Registration Exam Questions II

TOMORROW'S PHARMACIST

Welcome to the *Tomorrow's Pharmacist* series – helping you with your future career in pharmacy.

Like the journal, book titles under this banner are specifically aimed at pre-registration trainees and pharmacy students, to help them prepare for their future career. These books provide guidance on topics such as the interview and application process for the pre-registration year, the registration examination and future employment in a specific specialty.

The annual journal *Tomorrow's Pharmacist* will contain information and excerpts from the books in this series.

You can find more information on the journal at www.pjonline.com/tp.

Titles in the series so far include:

*The Pre-registration Interview: Preparation for the application process*

*Registration Exam Questions*

*MCQs in Pharmaceutical Calculations*

*Hospital Pre-registration Pharmacist Training*

# Registration Exam Questions II

## Nadia Bukhari

BPharm, MRPharmS, PG Cert Online Ed, PG Dip Pharm Prac, PG Dip Teaching Higher Ed

Student Support Manager and Pre-registration Coordinator School of Pharmacy, University of London, UK

## Naba Elsaid

MPharm, MRPharmS

Pre-registration Pharmacist Lecturer, Excel Pre-reg Training Classes, London, UK

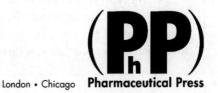

London • Chicago

**Published by the Pharmaceutical Press**

1 Lambeth High Street, London SE1 7JN, UK
1559 St. Paul Avenue, Gurnee, IL 60031, USA

© Royal Pharmaceutical Society of Great Britain 2011

(**PP**) is a trade mark of Pharmaceutical Press

Pharmaceutical Press is the publishing division of the Royal Pharmaceutical Society

First published 2011

Typeset by Thomson Digital, Noida, India
Printed in Great Britain by TJ International, Padstow, Cornwall
Index provided by Indexing Specialists, Hove, East Sussex, UK

ISBN 978 0 85369 976 7

A catalogue record for this book is available from the British Library

I would like to dedicate this book to my husband, Murtaza Bukhari, the wind beneath my wings. I love you not because of who you are, but because of who I am when I am with you −Nadia Bukhari.

I would like to dedicate this book to my wonderful parents, Fereedeh and Abed Elsaid −Naba Elsaid.

# Contents

Preface        ix
Acknowledgements        xi
About the author        xii
Abbreviations        xiii
How to use this book        xv

**Open book questions**                                    1

Simple completion questions                                1

Multiple completion questions                             18

Classification questions                                   29

Statement questions                                        38

**Open book answers**                                     47

Simple completion answers                                 47

Multiple completion answers                               56

Classification answers                                     64

Statement answers                                          74

**Closed book questions**                                 77

Simple completion questions                               77

Multiple completion questions                            109

Classification questions                                  122

Statement questions                                       130

**Closed book answers**                                    **137**

Simple completion answers                                   137

Multiple completion answers                                 149

Classification answers                                      157

Statement answers                                           165

**Calculation questions**                                  **169**

Simple completion  questions                                169

Multiple completion  questions                              178

Classification  questions                                   182

**Calculation answers**                                    **185**

Simple completion  answers                                  185

Multiple completion  answers                                190

Classification  answers                                     193

*Index*                                                     195

# Preface

After the success of the first edition of *Registration Exam Questions*, a decision was made to write a second book with even more questions than the first one.

This book is a bank of over 600 questions which are similar to the style of the registration examination. The questions are based on law and ethics, and clinical pharmacy and therapeutic aspects of the registration examination syllabus.

A new feature is a calculations chapter at the end of the book, with just over 50 practice open book questions.

After completing 4 years of study and graduating with a Master of Pharmacy (MPharm) degree, graduates are required to undertake training as a preregistration pharmacist before they can sit the registration examination.

Preregistration training is the period of employment on which graduates must embark and effectively complete before they can register as a pharmacist in Great Britain. In most cases it is a 1-year period following the pharmacy degree; for sandwich course students it is integrated within the undergraduate programme.

On successfully passing the registration examination, pharmacy graduates can register as a pharmacist in Great Britain.

The registration examination harmonises the testing of skills in practice during the preregistration year. It tests:

- knowledge
- the application of knowledge
- calculation
- time management
- managing stress
- comprehension
- recall
- interpretation
- evaluation.

There are two examination papers: an open book and a closed book paper. Questions are based on practice-based situations and are designed to test the thinking and knowledge that lie behind any action.

## EXAMINATION FORMAT

The registration examination consists of two papers:

1  closed book (no reference material can be used): 90 questions in 90 minutes (1.5 hours)
2  open book (three specified reference sources permitted):

- 80 questions in 150 minutes (2.5 hours)
- 60 non-calculation-style (recommended time for these 1.5 hours)
- 20 calculation-style (recommended time 1 hour).

The calculation-style questions are grouped together as a section of the paper.

The reference sources that the General Pharmaceutical Council permit for the registration examination are:

- *British National Formulary*
- *Drug Tariff for England and Wales or Drug Tariff for Scotland*
- *Medicines, Ethics and Practice Guide*

The registration examination is crucial for pharmacy graduates wishing to register in Great Britain.

Preparation is the key. This book cannot guarantee that you pass the registration examination; however, it can help you to practise the clinical pharmacy, law and ethics and calculation-type questions, all very important aspects of the registration examination, and, as they say, 'practice makes perfect'.

Good luck with the examination.

Nadia Bukhari, Naba Elsaid
January 2011

# Acknowledgements

The authors wish to acknowledge the support received from students and colleagues at the School of Pharmacy, University of London.

We especially thank our parents for their continuous support and encouragement.

We would like to express thanks to our editors at the Pharmaceutical Press, who have been very supportive, and especially to the publisher, Christina De Bono, and the senior development editor, Louise McIndoe, for their guidance.

# About the author

After qualifying, **Nadia Bukhari** worked as a pharmacy manager at Westbury Chemist, Streatham, London, for a year, after which she moved on to work for St Bartholomew's and the London NHS trust as a clinical pharmacist in surgery. It was at this time that Nadia developed an interest in teaching, as part of her role as a teacher practitioner for the School of Pharmacy, University of London.

Two and a half years later, she began working for the School of Pharmacy, University of London, as the preregistration coordinator for the school and the Master of Pharmacy (MPharm) programme manager. This position involved teaching therapeutics to MPharm students and assisting the academic director of studies.

Nadia's role has now evolved as the MPharm student support manager for the School as well as being the preregistration coordinator.

She has recently started one-to-one private tuition sessions as well as group tuition sessions for preregistration pharmacists covering all aspects of the examination syllabus. She has launched a new website, www.preregtuition.co.uk.

Recently Nadia has also taken on the role of subsection editor for pharmacy and clinical pharmacology for the *British Medical Journal*.

Nadia was a former question writer for the registration exam for 4 years, hence her interest in writing this book.

When first registered **Naba Elsaid** was employed as the pharmacist manager at one of Asda's busiest branches and was awarded two prizes for highest over-the-counter sales and maximum annual Medicines Use Review target achieved from 199 branches in the UK. She is now a lecturer at Excel Pre-reg, providing comprehensive seminars and support to pre-registration pharmacists.

# Abbreviations

| | |
|---|---|
| ACBS | Advisory Committee on Borderline Substances |
| ACE | angiotensin-converting enzyme |
| AV | arteriovenous |
| BMI | body mass index |
| BNF | *British National Formulary* |
| CD | controlled drug |
| CE | *conformité européenne* |
| CFC | chlorofluorocarbon |
| CHMP | Committee for Medicinal Products for Human Use |
| COX | cyclooxygenase |
| CSM | Committee on Safety of Medicines |
| CPD | continuous professional development |
| CYT | cytochrome |
| DNG | discount not given |
| DPF | Dental Practitioners' Formulary |
| EEA | European Economic Area |
| e/c | enteric-coated |
| eGFR | estimated glomerular filtration rate |
| GP | general practitioner |
| GP6D | glucose-6-phosphate dehydrogenase |
| GSL | general sales list |
| GTN | glyceryl trinitrate |
| HIV | human immunodeficiency virus |
| HRT | hormone replacement therapy |
| IBS | irritable bowel syndrome |
| IDA | industrial denatured alcohol |
| IM | intramuscular |
| IV | intravenous |
| IUD | intrauterine device |
| MAOI | monoamine oxidase inhibitor |
| MD | maximum single dose |
| MDD | maximum daily dose |
| MEP | *Medicines, Ethics and Practice Guide* |
| MHRA | Medicines and Healthcare products Regulatory Agency |

| | |
|---|---|
| MMR | measles, mumps and rubella |
| MR, m/r | modified release |
| MUPS | multiple-unit pellet system |
| MUR | Medicines Use Review |
| NHS | National Health Service |
| NSAIDs | non-steroidal anti-inflammatory drugs |
| OC | oral contraceptive |
| o.d. | omni die (every day) |
| o.m. | omni mane (every morning) |
| o.n. | omni nocte (every night) |
| OP | original pack |
| ORT | oral rehydration therapy |
| OTC | over-the-counter |
| P | pharmacy |
| PCT | primary care trust |
| PIL | patient information leaflet |
| PMR | patient medical record |
| POM | prescription-only medicine |
| POM-V | prescription-only medicine – veterinarian |
| POM-VPS | prescription-only medicine – veterinarian, pharmacist, suitably qualified person |
| PSA | prostate-specific antigen |
| PSNC | Pharmaceutical Services Negotiating Committee |
| q.d.s. | quater die sumendum (to be taken four times daily) |
| RPSGB | Royal Pharmaceutical Society of Great Britain |
| SARSS | Suspected Adverse Reaction Surveillance Scheme |
| SLS | selected list scheme |
| SOP | standard operating procedure |
| SPC | Summary of Product Characteristics |
| SSRI | selective serotonin reuptake inhibitor |
| TCA | tricyclic antidepressant |
| TSDA | trade-specific denatured alcohol |
| UTI | urinary tract infection |
| WHO | World Health Organization |

# How to use this book

The book is divided into two main sections: open book and closed book.

Each section has four different styles of multiple choice questions, which are also used in the registration examination: simple completion, multiple completion, classification and statements.

## SIMPLE COMPLETION QUESTIONS

Each of the questions or statements in this section is followed by five suggested answers. Select the best answer in each situation.

For example:
A patient on your ward has been admitted with a gastric ulcer, which is currently being treated. She has a history of arthritis and cardiac problems. Which of her drugs is most likely to have caused the gastric ulcer?

A  paracetamol
B  naproxen
C  furosemide
D  propranolol
E  codeine phosphate

## MULTIPLE COMPLETION QUESTIONS

Each one of the questions or incomplete statements in this section is followed by three responses. For each question, ONE or MORE of the responses is/are correct. Decide which of the responses is/are correct, then choose:

A    if 1, 2 and 3 are correct
B    if 1 and 2 only are correct
C    if 2 and 3 only are correct
D    if 1 only is correct
E    if 3 only is correct

For example:

A patient presents an FP10D to you.

Which of the below CANNOT be prescribed on this type of form?

1   ciprofloxacin
2   diclofenac
3   paracetamol

## CLASSIFICATION

In this section, for each numbered question, select the one lettered option that most closely corresponds to the answer. Within each group of questions each lettered option may be used once, more than once or not at all.

For example:

Which of the following vitamins:

1   can cause ocular defects in deficiency states?
2   is necessary for the production of blood-clotting factors?
3   prevents scurvy?
4   can be used for the treatment of rickets?

    A   vitamin A
    B   vitamin C
    C   vitamin D
    D   vitamin E
    E   vitamin K

## STATEMENTS

The questions in this section consist of a statement in the top row followed by a second statement beneath.

You need to:

decide whether the **first** statement is true or false

decide whether the **second** statement is true or false

Then choose:

A   if both statements are true and the second statement is **a correct explanation** of the first statement

B   if both statements are true but the second statement is **NOT a correct explanation** of the first statement

C   if the first statement is true but the second statement is false

D   if the first statement is false but the second statement is true

E   if both statements are false

For example:

**First statement**

*Microgynon* is an example of a combined oral contraceptive pill

**Second statement**

Combined pills contain oestrogen and testosterone

The closed book questions should be attempted without using any references sources, as you would for the examination.

The open book questions should be attempted with the Society's permitted reference sources for the registration examination, which are:

- *British National Formulary* (BNF)
- *Drug Tariff for England and Wales* or *Drug Tariff for Scotland*
- *Medicines, Ethics and Practice Guide* (MEP)

Answers to the questions are at the end of the open book and closed book sections. Brief explanations or a suitable reference for sourcing the answer are given, to aid understanding and to facilitate learning.

Important: This text refers to the editions of the BNF, Drug Tariff and MEP that were current when the text was written. Please always consult the LATEST version for the most up-to-date information.

# Open book questions

Nadia Bukhari, Naba Elsaid

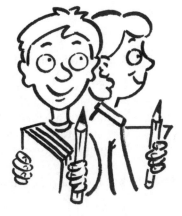

## SIMPLE COMPLETION QUESTIONS

Each of the questions or statements in this section is followed by five suggested answers. Select the best answer in each situation.

1   Which of the following should be completely avoided in pregnancy?

    **A**   tibolone
    **B**   levonorgestrel
    **C**   ferrous fumarate
    **D**   magnesium sulphate
    **E**   metoclopramide

2   Which of the following should *not* be given in severe hepatic impairment?

    **A**   vigabatrin
    **B**   telithromycin
    **C**   pegvisomant
    **D**   acetylsalicylic acid
    **E**   amisulpride

3   Which of the following should be avoided in renal impairment?

    **A**   verteporfin
    **B**   methysergide
    **C**   capreomycin
    **D**   nystatin
    **E**   mercaptopurine

4   Which of the following is *not* a black dot interaction?

    **A**   ritonavir + carbemazepine
    **B**   quinine + moxifloxacin
    **C**   ibuprofen + prednisolone
    **D**   memantine + amantadine
    **E**   lithium + arsenic trioxide

5   Which of the following is the trade name for leflunomide?

    **A**   *Seractil*
    **B**   *Arava*
    **C**   *Prostap SR*
    **D**   *Prograf*
    **E**   *Syntocinon*

6   Which of the following has the trade name *Integrilin*?

    **A**   eptifibatide
    **B**   omalizumab
    **C**   quinapril
    **D**   urokinase
    **E**   nitrazepam

7   Which of the following is a black dot interaction?

    **A**   tadalafil + fosamprenavir
    **B**   oral typhoid vaccine + tinidazole
    **C**   venlafaxine + moclobemide
    **D**   primidone + alcohol
    **E**   nicorandil + amitriptyline

8   Which of the following are the correct reconstitution directions for ciclosporin IV?

    **A**   Dissolve in 1 mL water for injections
    **B**   Reconstitute each vial with 12 mL water for injections
    **C**   Dilute to a concentration of 50 mg in 40 mL
    **D**   Reconstitute with 40 mL infusion fluid
    **E**   May be administered undiluted

9    Which of the following is not given in the BNF as a method of administering?

    **A**    intramuscular injection
    **B**    intermittent intravenous infusion (in glucose 5% over 30 minutes)
    **C**    slow intravenous injection
    **D**    continuous subcutaneous infusion
    **E**    intermittent intravenous infusion (in sodium chloride 0.9% over 30 minutes)

10   Which of the following is a high-energy fat supplement?

    **A**    *Protifar*
    **B**    *Energivit*
    **C**    *Caloreen*
    **D**    *SOS*
    **E**    *Polycal*

11   Which of the following is a nutritional supplement containing less than 1.5 kcal/mL and 5 g or more protein/100 mL?

    **A**    *Fortijuce*
    **B**    *Provide Xtra* juice drink
    **C**    *Ensure*
    **D**    *Resource* fruit
    **E**    *Oral Impact*

12   Which of the following is a side-effect for tibolone?

    **A**    anaemia
    **B**    seizures
    **C**    amnesia
    **D**    lethargy
    **E**    myocardial infarction

13   Which of the following should be used with caution in severe renal impairment?

    **A**    zotepine
    **B**    rotigotine
    **C**    abciximab
    **D**    iloprost
    **E**    sitaxentan sodium

14  Which of the following should be avoided in hepatic impairment?

    A   methysergide
    B   mebendazole
    C   corifollitropin alfa
    D   crotamiton
    E   propofol

15  Which of the following should be avoided in breast-feeding?

    A   protamine
    B   tinzaparin
    C   sodium valproate
    D   carboprost
    E   polysaccharide–iron complex

16  Which of the following is not known to be harmful whilst breast-feeding?

    A   anagrelide
    B   ergocalciferol
    C   adalimumab
    D   intrauterine progesterone-only system
    E   podophyllotoxin

17  Which of the following is known to be teratogenic?

    A   cyproterone acetate
    B   thalidomide
    C   cetuximab
    D   somatropin
    E   telbivudine

18  Which of the following is considered a black dot interaction?

    A   aspirin + metoclopramide
    B   nitrazepam + captopril
    C   olanzapine + fluvoxamine
    D   bleomycin + phenytoin
    E   carbamezepine + theophylline

19 Which of the following is a preparation that is monitored intensively by the MHRA?

    A   *Erbitux*
    B   *Targretin*
    C   *MUSE*
    D   *Intrinsa*
    E   *Fosamax*

20 Which of the following is the correct cautionary and advisory label for quetiapine?

    A   ... with or after food
    B   Warning. May cause drowsiness. If affected do not drive or operate machinery. Avoid alcoholic drink
    C   To be spread thinly ...
    D   ... with plenty of water
    E   Warning. May cause drowsiness

21 Which of the following is the correct cautionary and advisory label for gemfibrozil?

    A   ... sucked or chewed
    B   ... with or after food
    C   ... half to one hour before food
    D   ... dissolved under the tongue
    E   ... with plenty of water

22 Which of the following has the trade name *Tazocin*?

    A   co-fluampicil
    B   cefadroxil
    C   teicoplanin
    D   piperacillin with tazobactam
    E   cidofovir

23 Hepatitis is a side-effect of riluzole. It can occur in:

    A   1 in 10 individuals
    B   1 in 100 individuals
    C   1 in 500 individuals
    D   1 in 10 000 individuals
    E   less than 1 in 10 000 individuals

24 Which one of the following supplements should not be taken on the same day as alendronic acid?

    A    vitamin A
    B    vitamin B
    C    vitamin C
    D    calcium
    E    magnesium

25 Which of the following bacteria are Gram-positive:

    A    *Salmonella*
    B    *Shigella*
    C    *Pseudomonas*
    D    *Clostridium difficile*
    E    *Neisseria*

26 Which of the following is not a symptom of hypoglycaemia?

    A    sweating
    B    confusion
    C    anxiety or irritability
    D    polydipsia
    E    convulsions

27 Which of the following is *not* a side-effect of *Bricanyl Turbohaler*?

    A    fine tremor of the hands
    B    sleep disturbances
    C    headache
    D    collapse
    E    arthralgia

28 Which of the following preparations contains a high sodium content?

    A    *Alu-Cap* capsules
    B    *Maalox* suspension
    C    Aromatic magnesium carbonate oral suspension
    D    *Altacite Plus* suspension
    E    *Asilone* suspension

29  Which of the following HRT preparations would be suitable for a 54-year-old woman who has had a hysterectomy and does not suffer from endometriosis?

  A   *Premique*
  B   *Elleste-Duet*
  C   *Trisequens*
  D   *Nuvelle*
  E   *Zumenon*

30  Which one of the following products is *not* licensed as a medical device for use in the UK?

  A   *Medi-Test* protein 2
  B   *Nebuchamber* with child mask
  C   *Neocate Active*
  D   *Otovent* autoinflation for glue ear
  E   *Vitrex Soft* lancets

31  Which one of the following appliances is allowed to be prescribed on NHS prescriptions?

  A   *Accutrend* blood glucose meter
  B   *Bonjela* teether and gel pack
  C   *Bug Buster* kit
  D   centigrade thermometer
  E   *Glucolet 2* device

32  Which one of the following catheters attracts a fee of £3.40?

  A   *Scott* polythene catheter for girls
  B   *SpeediCath Control* male ordinary cylindrical catheter single use
  C   *Bard Reliacath* plastic male ordinary cylindrical catheter
  D   *Bard Biocath* hydrogel coated Foley catheter – two-way for long-term use in an adult male
  E   *Emteva* intermittent catheter with finger grip and lid

33   Dr F calls you to ask about a product which can be given to a patient who has hypoglycaemia. Which one of the following products can you recommend?

    **A**   *Foodlink Complete*
    **B**   *Jevity Plus*
    **C**   *KetoCal*
    **D**   *Pro-Cal*
    **E**   *Vita-Bite*

34   Which one of the following appliances *cannot* be prescribed on NHS FP10P forms?

    **A**   *Reflexions* flat spring vaginal contraceptive diaphragm
    **B**   *Allevyn Cavity* tubular dressing 9 × 2.5 cm
    **C**   *Lyclear Spray Away* pack
    **D**   *Balneum* bath oil
    **E**   *Aviva* biosensor strips

35   Which one of the following drugs will be reimbursed based on the listed brand price even if the generic is supplied?

    **A**   lorazepam 2.5 mg tablets
    **B**   sodium valproate 200 mg gastro-resistant tablets
    **C**   emulsifying wax
    **D**   raloxifene 60 mg tablets
    **E**   triclofos 500 mg/5 mL oral solution

36   Mrs J is a 58-year-old woman who is not exempt from paying NHS prescription charges. She presents an NHS prescription for the following items:

    Dilzem XL 180 mg capsules 1 × 28
    Tritace titration pack 1 × OP
    Scholl class II thigh stockings × 1 pair
How many prescription charges is she required to pay?

    **A**   2 charges
    **B**   3 charges
    **C**   4 charges
    **D**   5 charges
    **E**   7 charges

37  None of the following patients are exempt from paying NHS prescription charges. Which one of them will only pay *one* prescription charge?

    **A**   a woman with a prescription for knee caps (one-way stretch) 1 pair

    **B**   a woman with a prescription for *Migraleve* complete tablets

    **C**   a man with a prescription for *Biotene Oralbalance* dry mouth system

    **D**   a woman with a prescription for *Niaspan* MR titration pack

    **E**   a man with a prescription for prednisolone 1 mg tablets and prednisolone 2.5 mg e/c tablets

38  Mrs A is not exempt from paying NHS prescription charges. She presents you with the following prescription:

Compression hosiery class II
Thigh-length stocking circular knit (made to measure)
Mitte × 2 pairs
Suspender belt ×1
Suspenders ×2

How many prescription charges will you take from her?

    **A**   3
    **B**   4
    **C**   5
    **D**   6
    **E**   7

39  Which one of the following packs should *not* be split or broken?

    **A**   azithromycin 200 mg/5 mL oral suspension
    **B**   chalk powder
    **C**   coconut oil
    **D**   galantamine 8 mg tablets
    **E**   zuclopenthixol 2 mg tablets

40  Which one of the following items on a prescription should be endorsed with the pack size and brand name (or manufacturer's/wholesaler's name) in order to obtain the correct reimbursement fees?

    **A**   adapalene 0.1% gel
    **B**   dexketoprofen 25 mg tablets
    **C**   menthol 0.5% in aqueous cream
    **D**   cade oil liquid
    **E**   vancomycin 250 mg capsules

41  Broken bulk can be claimed on all of the following products except:

   A   dimeticone 22%/benzalkonium chloride 0.1% cream
   B   castor oil liquid
   C   fluticasone 0.05% cream
   D   menthol 0.5% in aqueous cream
   E   ginger syrup

42  An NHS prescription containing which one of the following items can be dispensed?

   A   *Codis* soluble tablets
   B   *Ozium* 3000
   C   *Delph* sun lotion SPF30
   D   *Microalbustix* strips
   E   Benzoin inhalation BP

43  Which one of the following items can be supplied under the NHS?

   A   *Clever Chek* strips
   B   *Glucoject No-dol* 30 gauge lancets
   C   *HumaPen Luxura* 3 mL reusable pen
   D   *Ketodiastix* strips
   E   *Rosidal K* short stretch compression bandage

44  Study the following extract from an NHS prescription issued to Mr Y by his GP to prevent him contracting influenza:

   Oseltamivir 75 mg capsules
   As directed
   Mitte × 1 OP

   How does the GP need to amend the prescription so that the pharmacy will be reimbursed for this prescription?

   A   The prescription should be referenced 'DNG'
   B   The prescription should be referenced 'ACBS'
   C   The prescription should be referenced 'SLS'
   D   The prescription should be referenced 'PNC'
   E   The total quantity must be specified in both words and figures

**45** Which one of the following is used in food as a colourant?

    **A**   sucrose
    **B**   rifampicin
    **C**   triamterene
    **D**   Ponceau 4R
    **E**   benzalkonium chloride

**46** Which one of the following drugs is contraindicated in a woman who is 23 weeks pregnant?

    **A**   carnitine
    **B**   citalopram
    **C**   dacarbazine
    **D**   oxycodone hydrochloride
    **E**   clindamycin

**47** To which one of the following customers (assuming there are no other contraindications) can *Tagamet* 100 be sold?

    **A**   a 13-year-old boy
    **B**   a 27-year-old female who is stabilised on phenytoin
    **C**   a 35-year-old man who is taking warfarin
    **D**   a 17-year-old boy who has heartburn only at night
    **E**   a 30-year-old female who is pregnant

**48** A woman, who has been on indapamide for 4 years, tells you about an 'unusual side-effect' which she suspects to be a result of her medication. Which one of the following adverse effects should be reported to the MHRA?

    **A**   postural hypotension
    **B**   gout
    **C**   headache
    **D**   visual disturbances
    **E**   infertility

**49** Which one of the following is considered to have a high risk of causing haemolysis in patients with G6PD deficiency?

    **A**   trimethoprim
    **B**   quinine
    **C**   nitrofurantoin
    **D**   phenytoin
    **E**   vitamin K

50  Which one of the following drugs is best administered at night?

>  A   *Imdur*
>  B   xipamide
>  C   paliperidone
>  D   *Pripsen* for a child
>  E   *Zimovane*

51  Mrs J, who is 37, comes into your pharmacy to discuss a symptom which she has recently developed that is worrying her. She is experiencing excessive daytime sleepiness and last week, whilst she was discussing a project with her colleague, she suddenly fell asleep. She also has consti-pation. Which of the following is the most likely cause for this?

>  A   *Lamictal* tablets
>  B   work stress
>  C   *Mirapexin* tablets
>  D   *Ledermycin* capsules
>  E   cluster headache

52  With which of the following drugs should patients be told to stop taking their medication and report to their doctor if they develop increased urinary frequency, nocturia, urgency, pain on urinating or blood in their urine?

>  A   duloxetine
>  B   *Flomaxtra XL*
>  C   *Hygroton*
>  D   tiaprofenic acid
>  E   *AT-10*

53  Which one of the following antacids does *not* contain a low $Na^+$ content?

>  A   hydrotalcite suspension
>  B   *Altacite Plus* suspension
>  C   *Topal* tablets
>  D   *Gaviscon Advance* tablets
>  E   *Maalox* suspension

54  Which one of the following drugs is unsafe for use in acute porphyria?

    **A**   ramipril
    **B**   rosuvastatin
    **C**   fluoxetine
    **D**   diazoxide
    **E**   nandrolone

55  Mrs H has an estimated glomerular filteration rate of 35 mL/min/1.73 m². Which one of the following drugs can be supplied to her?

    **A**   atenolol 100 mg o.d.
    **B**   codeine 60 mg q.d.s.
    **C**   moxonidine 200 micrograms o.m.
    **D**   methysergide 1 mg o.n.
    **E**   tetracycline 250 mg q.d.s.

56  Mr K has been prescribed *Etrivex* shampoo to use for his psoriasis. How long can he continue to use this preparation?

    **A**   5 days
    **B**   10 days
    **C**   1 week
    **D**   2 weeks
    **E**   4 weeks

57  Which one of the following is *not* an established side-effect of *Lipostat*?

    **A**   rhabdomyolysis
    **B**   jaundice
    **C**   weight gain
    **D**   hair loss
    **E**   nocturia

58  Which one of the following classes of antidepressants is the first-line treatment for depression?

    **A**   tricyclic antidepressant drugs
    **B**   monoamine oxidase inhibitors
    **C**   selective serotonin reuptake inhibitors
    **D**   serotonin and noradrenaline reuptake inhibitors
    **E**   selective reuptake inhibitors of noradrenaline

59 With which of the following drugs are extrapyramidal symptoms more likely to occur?

    A   aripiprazole
    B   clozapine
    C   haloperidol
    D   trifluoperazine
    E   olanzapine

60 Which one of the following is *not* a sign of iron poisoning?

    A   abdominal pain
    B   blood in the vomit
    C   nausea/vomitting
    D   rectal bleeding
    E   corneal microdeposits

61 Barbiturates are known to reduce the effects of many drugs. Which one of the following drugs has no known drug interaction with barbiturates?

    A   ciclosporin
    B   lercanidipine
    C   ibuprofen
    D   warfarin
    E   *Cilest*

62 Mrs A is allergic to aspirin. Which one of the following preparations can be supplied to her?

    A   *Synflex* tablets
    B   *Resprin* suppositories
    C   co-codaprin dispersible tablets
    D   *Remedeine* tablets
    E   *Flamasacard* capsules

63 Which one of the following is *not* a desirable feature of an oral rehydration therapy solution?

    A   It should enhance the absorption of water and electrolytes
    B   It should be simple to use in hospital and at home
    C   It should contain an acidic agent
    D   It should be slightly hypo-osmolar
    E   It should be palatable and acceptable, especially to children

64 You are asked about the strength of *Amias* tablets which a patient has taken. You are told that the tablets are white and scored. Which one of the following strengths has the patient been taking?

    A   2 mg
    B   4 mg
    C   8 mg
    D   16 mg
    E   32 mg

65 Which one of the following smooth-muscle relaxants *cannot* be sold to the public?

    A   *Colpermin* capsules
    B   *Buscopan*
    C   dicycloverine hydrochloride 20 mg tablets
    D   *Kolanticon* gel
    E   mebeverine hydrochloride 135 mg (MD) and 405 mg (MDD) for IBS

66 Which one of the following medications is *not* exempt from normal restrictions when administered parenterally for the purpose of saving a life?

    A   naloxone hydrochloride
    B   hydrocortisone
    C   adrenaline 1 mg/1 mL
    D   chlorphenamine
    E   acetylcysteine

67 In regard to the requirements for labelling of pharmacy medicines, which additional warning must appear on products containing hexachlorophane?

    A   Not to be used for babies
    B   Do not exceed the stated dose
    C   May cause drowsiness
    D   For external use only
    E   Keep out of the reach and sight of children

68 Which of the following is *not* a requirement for the recording of whole-sale supplies of prescription-only medicines?

    A    medicine's name, form, strength and quantity
    B    date of supply
    C    name and address of the purchaser
    D    the reason for the supply
    E    name and address of the patients

69 Which one of the following drugs requires the dose to be specified on the prescription?

    A    diazepam
    B    temazepam
    C    *Cosalgesic*
    D    atamestane
    E    benzfetamine

70 Which one of the following must be rendered 'irretrievable' before disposal?

    A    *Adalat* LA tablets
    B    *Andropatch*
    C    *Feminax Ultra*
    D    *Dormonoct* tablets
    E    *Oramorph* 10 mg/5 mL oral solution

71 A patient has run out of medication and has come into your pharmacy to request a supply to cover the bank holiday weekend. Which one of the following drugs *cannot* be supplied in this case?

    A    phenobarbital tablets
    B    insulin injection
    C    diazepam tablets
    D    *Frisium* tablets
    E    temazepam tablets

72 Which one of the following is *not* a legal requirement for the labelling of prescription-only medicines?

    A    medicinal form
    B    cautionary statements
    C    supplier's name
    D    date dispensed
    E    directions for use

73 In exceptional circumstances, a pharmacist may release confidential information to an authorised person. Release of confidential information should *not* be made to:

    **A**   HM coroner
    **B**   judge
    **C**   court order
    **D**   Crown prosecution officer
    **E**   verbal request from a police officer

*The answers for this section are on pp. 47–55.*

## MULTIPLE COMPLETION QUESTIONS

Each one of the questions or incomplete statements in this section is followed by three responses. For each question, ONE or MORE of the responses is/are correct. Decide which of the responses is/are correct, then choose:

A    if 1, 2 and 3 are correct
B    if 1 and 2 only are correct
C    if 2 and 3 only are correct
D    if 1 only is correct
E    if 3 only is correct

| Summary | | | | |
|---------|---------|-----------|--------|--------|
| A | B | C | D | E |
| 1, 2, 3 | 1, 2 only | 2, 3 only | 1 only | 3 only |

1   Which of the following is/are side-effects of voriconazole?

    1   jaundice
    2   hyperthyroidism
    3   nystagmus

2   Which of the following is/are safe to give in pregnancy?

    1   isophane insulin
    2   isoniazid
    3   benzylpenicillin

3   Which of the following is/are used for the treatment of non-Hodgkin's lymphoma?

    1   bleomycin
    2   doxorubicin
    3   idarubicin

4   Which of the following is/are not recommended in moderate renal impairment?

1   vardenafil
2   ganirelix
3   alendronic acid

5   Which of the following is/are indicated for treatment of alcohol dependence?

1   bupropion hydrochloride
2   nicotine
3   disulfiram

6   Which of the following is/are a caution with the treatment of rizatriptan?

1   elderly
2   pre-existing cardiac disease
3   anaemia

7   Which of the following may be prescribed for vitamin $B_6$ deficiency?

1   pyridoxine
2   ascorbic acid
3   ergocalciferol

8   Which of the following has/have a definite risk of haemolysis in G6PD-deficient individuals?

1   nitrofurantoin
2   ciprofloxacin
3   dapsone

9   Which of the following has/have a possible risk of haemolysis in G6PD-deficient individuals?

1   niridazole
2   quinine
3   probenecid

10   Which of the following has/have a definite risk of haemolysis in G6PD-deficient individuals?

1   pamaquin
2   chloroquine
3   quinine

11  Which of the following vaccines is/are *not* contraindicated in a patient with a known anaphylactic reaction to eggs?

1   MMR
2   yellow fever
3   tick-borne encephalitis

12  Class 1 graduated compression hosieries can be used for:

1   superficial varices
2   mild oedema
3   postthrombotic venous insufficiency

13  Which of the following preparations is/are prolonged-release formulations?

1   *Prograf*
2   *Modigraf*
3   *Advagraf*

14  Which of the following should patients be told to report promptly to their doctors?

1   nipple discharge in a 47-year-old man using finasteride 5 mg daily for male-pattern baldness
2   sore throat in a 38-year-old female using carbimazole 30 mg daily for hyperthyroidism
3   nocturia in a 57-year-old female receiving tiaprofenic acid 300 mg twice daily for rheumatic disease

15  Which of the following excipients could cause a fatal toxic syndrome in preterm neonates?

1   benzyl alcohol
2   poloxyl castor oil
3   propylene glycol

16  Which of the following drugs does/do not cause xerostomia?

1   hyoscine
2   clozapine
3   metoclopramide

17  Which of the following antimalarials is/are contraindicated in pregnancy?

1   doxycycline
2   chloroquine
3   proguanil

18  Malathion can be used to treat which of the following:

1   *Sarcoptes scabiei*
2   *Pediculus humanus capitis*
3   tinea pedis

19  Carbomer eye gel is available in different viscosities. Which of the following products contains carbomer 980?

1   *GelTears*
2   *Liposic*
3   *Liquivisc*

20  Which of the following is/are true in regard to the duties of the responsible pharmacist?

1   has a legal obligation to ensure safe and effective sale and supply of medicines
2   must display a notice at the premises showing name, registration number and hours of work
3   can leave the premises for a maximum of 1 hour in any 24-hour period

21  Which of the following medications is/are *not* licensed for over-the-counter supply to the following patients?

1   1% hydrocortisone cream (15 g tube) to a 9-year-old boy with mild eczema
2   4 weeks' supply of nizatidine for an 18-year-old with food-induced heartburn
3   5 days' supply of naproxen 250 mg tablets for the treatment of primary dysmenorrhoea in a 25-year-old woman

22  Which of the following is/are not subject to the Fluted Bottles Regulations 1978?

1   a 1 L bottle of carvacrol
2   eye or ear drops sold or supplied in a glass container
3   medicines used for research purposes

23 Which of the following conditions must be satisfied for a pharmacist to become a distributor of IDA and TSDA?

1 does not denature alcohol on the premises on which it is kept
2 deals or intends to deal wholesale in denatured alcohol
3 holds an excise licence

24 With respect to the record-keeping of POM-V and POM-VPS, which of the following apply/applies?

1 Records must be kept for a minimum of 5 years from the last entry
2 Entries must include the name, form and strength of the product
3 Entries must include the prescriber's identification number

25 Regarding medicines for veterinary use, which of the following statements is/are true?

1 A prescription for CD 2 or 3 drug (excluding temazepam) must specify the name and address of the person to whom the CD is to be delivered
2 A person who has food-producing animals must keep proof of obtaining any medicines for the animals
3 The sale/supply of any class of veterinary medicines from a registered pharmacy must be supervised by a pharmacist

26 Which of the following is/are monitored by the Suspected Adverse Reaction Surveillance Scheme (SARSS)?

1 adverse reactions to veterinary or human medicines in animals only
2 recent human exposure to a medically treated animal
3 suspected medicinal residues in the milk of treated cows

27 Regarding the emergency supply of prescription-only medicines, which of the following statements is/are false?

1 Supply can be made at the request of a doctor or a dentist (including EEA or Swiss prescribers)
2 Schedule 4 and 5 controlled drugs can be supplied at the request of UK authorised prescribers or at the request of patients
3 Supplies at the request of a prescriber require a prescription to be furnished within 24 hours

28 According to the Medicines Act 1968, a registered retail pharmacy can wholesale medicines to:

    1    another wholesaler
    2    primary care trust
    3    UK-registered vet

29 The Chemicals (Hazard Information and Packaging for Supply) Regulations 2002 require the following to appear on the label of a chemical before it is supplied:

    1    name, address and telephone number of the supplier
    2    both the risk and safety phrases
    3    the phrase 'warning: for external use only'

30 The following is/are legal prescription requirement(s) for diamorphine:

    1    It can be prescribed on an FP10MDA form by any prescriber for the treatment of addiction
    2    Private prescriptions must be on standardised forms and include the prescriber's registration number and the originals must be sent to the relevant NHS agency
    3    The direction 'one when required' or 'one as directed' is acceptable

31 The following applies/apply to requisitions for schedule 2 or 3 controlled drugs:

    1    They must be hand-written and state the reason for the request
    2    Practitioners have 72 hours in which to provide a requisition from the requested date
    3    It is good practice to use a standardised requisition form between community pharmacies

32 Regarding the following NHS prescription:

    Nabilone capsules 1 mg
    One to be taken as directed
    Mitte × 20 capsules

Which of the following statements is/are true?

    1    After taking all necessary measures, pharmacists can amend this prescription so that it contains the total quantity in both words and figures
    2    Pharmacies can accept patient-returned controlled drugs from residential care homes
    3    Destruction of nabilone as part of the pharmacy's own stock requires an authorised witness (e.g. accountable officer) to be present

33 Regarding the duties of the responsible pharmacist, which of the following statements is/are true?

1 The responsible pharmacist is legally responsible for the safe and effective sale and supply of all classes of medicines

2 *Denorex* shampoo (125 mL) does *not* need to be sold under the supervision of a pharmacist

3 P or POM products can only be sold under the supervision of a pharmacist even in the event of a pandemic

34 Which of the following statements is/are true regarding *Lanoxin* injection?

1 Water for injection is a suitable infusion fluid

2 Protect from light

3 To be administered over at least 2 hours

35 Which of the following statements is/are true regarding glyceryl trinitrate?

1 Short-acting tablets should be supplied in glass containers with a foil-lined cap and cotton wool wadding

2 Postural hypotension, throbbing headache and dizziness are common side-effects of this drug

3 Tolerance may develop in patients who are using *Deponit* patches

36 Which of the following statements is/are true with regard to adverse reaction reporting?

1 Adverse reactions to therapeutic agents (e.g. herbal products) or medical devices should be reported to the MHRA

2 Patients or their carers should report any adverse effects to NHS Direct

3 Report all suspected reactions for unlicensed medicines shown by the symbol (▼)

37 Which of the following symptoms should a patient who is taking carbimazole for hyperthyroidism be advised to report immediately?

1 taste disturbances

2 unexplained bruising

3 flu-like symptoms (e.g. sore throat)

38 Gabapentin may be used to treat which of the following conditions?

1 epilepsy

2 phantom limb pain

3 anxiety

39  Miss E, a lively teenager, gives you her prescription for *Roaccutane* capsules. As you hand over the medication to her she tells you, 'I can't wait for this weekend. My boyfriend's taking me camping in Wales'. What advice do you give her?

  1  Practise effective contraception while taking *Roaccutane* and for 1 month following treatment
  2  Avoid wax epilation
  3  Avoid UV light/sunlight and use sunscreen and emollient

40  During doctor–patient consultations, which of the following conditions must be reported to the proper officer of the local authority?

  1  food poisoning
  2  ophthalmia neonatorum
  3  whooping cough

41  Which of the following antibiotics can be used to treat community-acquired pneumonia of low severity?

  1  ceftazidime
  2  meropenem
  3  doxycycline

42  Miss C is allergic to iodine. Which of the following medications should she avoid?

  1  *Savlon* dry powder spray
  2  *Oxyzyme* hydrogel
  3  amiodarone tablets

43  The Yellow Card scheme is the system whereby adverse drug reactions are to be reported to the MHRA. Which of the following should be reported to the MHRA?

  1  adverse reactions to medical devices, including dental or surgical materials, intrauterine devices, X-ray contrast media and contact lens fluids
  2  all *serious* adverse reactions to established therapeutic agents, including over-the-counter, herbal, unlicensed or off-label products and vaccines
  3  any adverse reactions (including minor reactions) in children under the age of 19 years

44 When prescribing drugs for patients with renal impairment, which of the following statements is/are correct?

   1   Sensitivity to some drugs is increased even if elimination is unimpaired

   2   Drug dosages should be adjusted only to overweight patients

   3   Raised serum creatinine alone is a good indicator of renal impairment

45 Regarding the use of an antipsychotic in an emergency, which of the following statements is/are true?

   1   The intramuscular dose should be higher than the corresponding oral dose in highly active patients

   2   The prescription should specify the dose for each route and should not imply that the same dose can be given by mouth or by intramuscular injection

   3   The emergency dose should be reviewed on a daily basis

46 Regarding dexamfetamine poisoning and its treatment, which of the following statements is/are false?

   1   Amphetamines may cause excessive activity, hallucinations and coma

   2   Lorazepam can be used to treat the early signs of amphetamine poisoning

   3   Hypertension should be treated immediately with clonidine hydrochloride

47 Mrs J has recently been prescribed *Asasantin Retard* for the secondary prevention of ischaemic stroke. Regarding the packaging of *Asasantin Retard*, which of the following is/are true?

   1   Capsules must not be transferred to another container

   2   Capsules should not be broken and must be swallowed whole

   3   Unused capsules should be discarded 8 weeks after first opening the container

48 Which of the following preparations is/are likely to reduce the effectiveness of latex condoms during sexual intercourse?

   1   baby oil

   2   arachis oil enema

   3   *Vaseline*

49  Which of the following items is/are allowed to be ordered on an FP10D form?

    1   *Orabase* paste
    2   saliva *Orthana*
    3   co-codamol 8/500 tablets

50  Which of the following contraceptives is/are exempt from payment on an NHS FP10 form?

    1   *Katya*
    2   *Gygel*
    3   *FemCap* soft silicone cap

51  Regarding additional fees, which of the following statements is/are true?

    1   Home delivery of incontinence products attracts an additional fee
    2   All category E products must be endorsed with 'ED' to obtain the specified additional fee
    3   Dispensing any drug in schedules 2, 3 or 4 part I will attract the specified additional fee

52  For which of the following items should a pharmacist endorse 'DNG' to avoid discount being removed in respect of NHS prescription reimbursement?

    1   unlicensed POM ordered on a named-patient basis
    2   controlled drugs in schedules 1, 2 and 3
    3   *Hepsera* 10 mg tablets

53  Which of the following drugs prescribed on an FP10D/GP14 (Scotland) prescription would lead you to contact the prescriber for an alternative?

    1   sodium fusidate ointment
    2   aciclovir 800 mg tablets
    3   doxycycline 50 mg capsules

54  Regarding claiming out-of-pocket expenses, which of the following statements is/are true?

    1   can be claimed on staff working hours
    2   cannot be claimed on items in part IXA or IXR
    3   prescriptions with special items should be referenced with 'XP' and include details on the amount being claimed and the reason for the claim

55 Which of the following statements, regarding the use of *Spiriva*, is/are true?

   1    One puff of *Spiriva Respimat* solution is equivalent to 5 micrograms tiotropium

   2    *Spiriva* should be used with caution in those with an eGFR of less than $50 \, \text{mL/min}/1.73 \, \text{m}^2$

   3    The most common side-effect of this bronchodilator is dry mouth

56 Which of the following statements, regarding prednisolone, is/are true?

   1    5 mg prednisolone is equivalent to 10 mg hydrocortisone, with respect to the anti-inflammatory activity of these steroids

   2    Prednisolone has more mineralocorticoid activity than hydrocortisone

   3    Side-effects of prednisolone include diabetes and osteoporosis

57 Regarding antidepressant drugs, which of the following statements is/are false?

   1    The dose of antidepressant drugs should be reduced over a 2-week period prior to stopping therapy

   2    SSRIs are better tolerated in overdose than TCAs

   3    Anxiolytics are used with caution in patients suffering from depression

58 Which of the following preparations can be sold to the public?

   1    2% sodium cromoglicate 10 mL eye drops for the treatment of acute seasonal allergic conjunctivitis

   2    0.1% lodoxamide eye drops to an 38-year-old man suffering from allergic conjunctivitis

   3    *Beconase Hayfever* nasal spray to a 25-year-old woman, for the prevention of allergic rhinitis

59 Which of the following is/are correct regarding diagnostic tools?

   1    Fluorescein sodium is used for locating a damaged area within the cornea

   2    *Diabur Test-5000* is used to diagnose *Helicobacter pylori* bacterial infection

   3    Tetracosactide is used to diagnose adrenal insufficiency (by a rise in the plasma concentration of cortisol after its administration)

*The answers for this section are on pp. 56–63.*

## CLASSIFICATION QUESTIONS

In this section, for each numbered question, select the one lettered option that most closely corresponds to the answer. Within each group of questions each lettered option may be used once, more than once or not at all.

Questions 1–5 concern the following drugs:

A   ondansetron
B   clonidine
C   acemetacin
D   brinzolamide
E   dantrolene

Which of the above:

1  is indicated for raised intraocular pressure?
2  is considered less suitable for prescribing by the Joint Formulary Committee?
3  can be given in moderate or severe hepatic impairment with a maximum dose of 8 mg daily?
4  is indicated for pain in rheumatic disease?
5  is prescribed for the prevention of recurrent migraine?

Questions 6–10 concern the following drugs:

A   colistin
B   valaciclovir
C   danazol
D   rimexolone
E   flutamide

Which of the above:

6   is indicated for advanced prostate cancer?
7   may be prescribed for the treatment of infertility?
8   may cause pelious hepatitis as a side-effect?
9   is indicated for herpes zoster?
10  is contraindicated in patients with myasthenia gravis?

Questions 11–20 concern the following drugs:

A   *Indivina*
B   *Axorid*
C   *Morhulin*
D   *Dalmane*
E   *Resolor*

Which of the above:

11   is monitored intensively by the MHRA?
12   contains the hormone oestradiol?
13   is indicated for mild inflammation?
14   is a barrier preparation?
15   is a blacklisted item on an NHS prescription?
16   is a hypnotic?
17   is indicated for constipation in women?
18   is indicated for hormone replacement therapy for women with an intact uterus?
19   contains omeprazole as part of its formulation?
20   contains cod liver oil and can be used for minor wounds?

Questions 21–30 concern the following drugs:

A   *Mycobutin*
B   *Neo-Mercazole*
C   *Haleraid*
D   *Plavix*
E   *Marevan*

Which of the above:

21   is an anticoagulant?
22   requires regular monitoring of prothrombin time?
23   requires immediate medical attention if a sore throat develops?
24   may colour the urine red/orange?
25   is a blacklisted item on an NHS prescription?
26   has a daily dose of 75 mg?
27   antagonises the effects of vitamin K?
28   can be used in conjunction with *Seretide* inhalers?
29   is manufactured by Amdipharm?
30   are red-brown capsules?

Questions 31–40 concern the following drugs:

    A  *Tritace*
    B  *Inderal-LA*
    C  *Securon*
    D  *Lescol*
    E  *Sabril*

Which of the above:

**31**  should be discontinued if rhabdomyolysis occurs?
**32**  is to be used with caution in first-degree AV block?
**33**  may cause coldness of the extremities?
**34**  is classed as an ACE inhibitor?
**35**  is associated with visual field defects?
**36**  is manufactured by Astra Zeneca?
**37**  should be swallowed whole and not chewed?
**38**  comes as red 5 mg tablets?
**39**  comes as a sachet and should be dissolved in water immediately before taking?
**40**  may reduce uterine blood flow with fetal hypoxia in pregnancy?

Questions 41–50 concern the following drugs:

    A  clomethiazole
    B  ethosuximide
    C  calcitonin
    D  dasatinib
    E  lidocaine

Which of the above:

**41**  is contraindicated in alcohol-dependent patients who continue to drink?
**42**  may cause suicide ideation as a side-effect?
**43**  has the brand name *Miacalcic*?
**44**  is extracted from salmon?
**45**  is a tyrosine kinase inhibitor?
**46**  is indicated for acute lymphoblastic leukaemia?
**47**  can be used for ventricular arrhythmias?
**48**  increases the risk of side-effects with hepatic impairment?
**49**  may increase cerebral sensitivity in renal impairment?
**50**  is used in typical absence seizures?

Questions 51–60 concern the following drugs:

A   clozapine
B   erdosteine
C   dipyridamole
D   enoxaparin
E   sitaxentan sodium

Which of the above:

**51**   is a low-molecular-weight heparin?
**52**   in modified-release form should be dispensed in the original container?
**53**   does the manufacturer advise a maximum dose of 300 mg daily in mild hepatic impairment?
**54**   may cause fatal myocarditis?
**55**   should be withdrawn over 1–2 weeks?
**56**   requires blood monitoring every week for the first 18 weeks of treatment?
**57**   needs to be ordered from Polarspeed?
**58**   costs £1540 for a pack of 28 tablets?
**59**   is prescribed for the prophylaxis of pulmonary embolism?
**60**   should be avoided if a patient's eGFR is <25 mL/min/173 m$^2$?

Questions 61 and 62 concern the following drug combinations:

A   captopril and amiloride
B   verapamil and propranolol
C   glucosamine and warfarin
D   levothyroxine and iron
E   digoxin and amiodarone

Which of the above combination of drugs:

**61**   can cause an increased risk of severe hyperkalaemia?
**62**   should be taken at least 2 hours apart?

Questions 63–65 concern the following minerals:

A   calcium
B   magnesium
C   zinc
D   phosphate
E   fluoride

Which of the above:

**63** may be depleted in patients suffering from severe diabetic ketoacidosis?
**64** is the first-line treatment for seizures in women suffering from eclampsia?
**65** can cause hypocalcaemia when given in excessive doses?

Questions 66 and 67 concern the following controlled drugs:

    **A** clenbuterol
    **B** diazepam
    **C** hexobarbitone
    **D** phenobarbital
    **E** quinalbarbitone

Which of the above:

**66** has no restriction on possession when contained in its medicinal form?
**67** requires safe custody?

Questions 68 and 69 concern the following medicines:

    **A** borotannic complex 9%
    **B** diamorphine
    **C** methylprednisolone
    **D** nitrazepam
    **E** phytomenadione

Which of the above may be:

**68** administered by a registered chiropodist to his/her patient?
**69** supplied by a dentist to his/her patient?

Questions 70 and 71 concern the following:

    **A** 50%
    **B** 5%
    **C** 0.5%
    **D** 0.05%
    **E** 0.25%

Which of the above strengths reclassifies the following POMs to P medicines?

70  aciclovir used to treat a cold sore on the lips
71  clobetasone cream for a 14-year-old with a small patch of dermatitis on her arm

Questions 72 and 73 concern the following medicines:

    A   temazepam
    B   brotizolam
    C   *Codipar* caplets
    D   LSD
    E   metopon

Which of the above:

72  requires a home office licence for the manufacture, possession or supply?
73  does *not* require a licence for import or export?

Questions 74 and 75 concern the following medicines:

    A   *Acumed* patch
    B   *Mandanol* 32 tablets
    C   *Cystofem* sachets
    D   *Daktarin* (Janssen-Cilag) oral gel
    E   *Nylax* with senna 30 tablets

Which of the above can be sold:

74  from a non-pharmacy retail outlet?
75  only from a registered pharmacy under the supervision of a registered pharmacist?

Questions 76 and 77 concern the following drugs:

    A   *Xarelto* tablets
    B   *Welldorm* tablets
    C   *Adcal D$_3$* effervescent tablets
    D   *Diconal* tablets
    E   penicillamine tablets

Which of the above contains the following advisory labels:

76  To be taken with plenty of water?

77  Do not take indigestion remedies or medicines containing iron or zinc at the same time of day as this medicine?

Questions 78 and 79 concern the following topical preparations:

    A    *Dermovate*
    B    *Eumovate*
    C    *Synalar*
    D    *Locorten-Vioform*
    E    *Grisol AF*

Which of the above:

78  stains the skin and clothes?
79  is classed as a potent corticosteroid preparation?

Questions 80 and 81 concern the following medications:

    A    *Convulex* capsules
    B    *Roaccutane* capsules
    C    *Locorten-Vioform* ear drops
    D    *Utinor* tablets
    E    *Dostinex* tablets

Which of the above:

80  should not be given to patients who are allergic to peanuts?
81  should be dispensed in its original container?

Questions 82 and 83 concern the following preparations:

    A    *Acnamino MR* capsules
    B    *Strattera* capsules
    C    *Moviprep* oral powder
    D    *Gygel* gel
    E    *Antepsin*

Which of the above:

82  should be swallowed whole with plenty of fluid while sitting or standing?
83  contains E200 and E1520?

Questions 84 and 85 concern the following drugs:

    A   *Fosavance* tablets
    B   *Losec MUPS* tablets
    C   *Protium* tablets
    D   risperidone orodispersible tablets
    E   *Utrogestan* capsules

Which of the above:

84   should be placed on the tongue, allowed to dissolve and swallowed?
85   can be dispersed in water or mixed with fruit juice or yoghurt?

Questions 86 and 87 concern the following drugs:

    A   ciclosporin
    B   fosinopril sodium
    C   acitretin
    D   tranylcypromine
    E   tinidazole

Select one drug which, when taken with:

86   grapefruit juice, increases the risk of toxicity
87   alcohol, increases the risk of teratogenicity in women of child-bearing
     potential

Questions 88 and 89 concern the following:

    A   *Chloromycetin Redidrops*
    B   sucralfate suspension
    C   *Dalmane* capsules
    D   *Lotemax* eye drops
    E   *Cholestagel* tablets

Which of the above:

88   may form a hard indigestible mass of material?
89   should not be used for longer than 14 days?

Questions 90 and 91 concern the following proprietary preparations:

    A   *Orelox* tablets
    B   *Codalax* oral suspension
    C   *Myfortic* tablets
    D   *Dovonex* cream
    E   *Psorin* ointment

Which of the above products requires the following advisory labels?

**90**  To be spread thinly
**91**  Take at regular intervals. Complete the prescribed course unless otherwise directed

Questions 92 and 93 concern the following proprietary preparations:

    A   *Accupro* 20 mg tablets
    B   *Angitil* SR 90 mg capsules
    C   *Rifadin* syrup
    D   *Tilade* CFC-free inhaler
    E   *Uriben* suspension

Which of the above products is:

**92**  mint-flavoured?
**93**  brown in colour?

Questions 94 and 95 concern the following preparations:

    A   *Avodart* capsules
    B   *Duofilm* paint
    C   *Fasigyn* tablets
    D   *Rowachol* capsules
    E   *Zerit* capsules

Which of the above carries the following cautionary labels?

**94**  Caution flammable: keep away from fire or flames
**95**  Warning. Avoid alcoholic drink

*The answers for this section are on pp. 64–73.*

## STATEMENT QUESTIONS

The questions in this section consist of a statement in the top row followed by a second statement beneath.

You need to:

decide whether the **first** statement is true or false

decide whether the **second** statement is true or false

Then choose:

A    if both statements are true and the second statement is **a correct explanation** of the first statement

B    if both statements are true but the second statement is **NOT a correct explanation** of the first statement

C    if the first statement is true but the second statement is false

D    if the first statement is false but the second statement is true

E    if both statements are false

1    **First statement**

Expired *OxyContin* tablets can be kept in the controlled drug cabinet with the in-date stock

**Second statement**

The Home Office has advised that schedule 2 controlled drugs must be denatured before being put in waste containers

2    **First statement**

A registered midwife may possess pentazocine

**Second statement**

A midwife is required to keep a record of pentazocine

3    **First statement**

Pharmacists may keep their controlled drug records electronically

**Second statement**

Electronic records must be capable of printing or displaying the strength and form of the controlled drug

4  **First statement**

It is a legal requirement to sign on collection of a schedule 2 controlled drug

**Second statement**

It is a legal requirement to ascertain who the person collecting the schedule 2 controlled drug is

5  **First statement**

It is a legal requirement that no more than 30 days' supply is made of a schedule 3 controlled drug

**Second statement**

If more than 30 days is prescribed, prescribers will need to justify the basis of prescribing more than the requirement

6  **First statement**

Cannabis is a schedule 1 controlled drug

**Second statement**

Pharmacists may possess cannabis if they have a licence from the Home Office

7  **First statement**

The Home Secretary has the power to make a direction against a practitioner prohibiting him or her from prescribing controlled drugs

**Second statement**

This bill was passed under the Misuse of Drugs Act 1971

8  **First statement**

The Medicines Order 1979 prohibits the sale or supply of any medicinal product containing chloroform

**Second statement**

A supply may be made by a doctor who has prepared the medicinal product for a patient

9 **First statement**

*Creon* granules is a pharmacy-only product

**Second statement**

The Order of Malta Ambulance Corps can obtain this in wholesale from the pharmacy

10 **First statement**

A paramedic may administer certain parenteral medicines

**Second statement**

Diazepam 5 mg/mL emulsion for injection can be administered by a paramedic

11 **First statement**

In Scotland, the Waste Management Licensing Amendment Regulations 2006 allow registered pharmacies to accept patient-returned medication from patients or individuals

**Second statement**

Pharmacies in Scotland may accept returned waste from child care agencies

12 **First statement**

Pharmacists can sell plano cosmetic contact lenses without the supervision of a registered optician

**Second statement**

Pharmacists wishing to sell zero-powered contact lenses should do so in accordance with the relevant legal requirements contained within the Opticians Act 1984

13 **First statement**

Completely denatured alcohol is suitable for general domestic use

**Second statement**

Pharmacists deal with this type of alcohol

14 **First statement**

*Salmosan* can be dispensed by a registered pharmacy premises

**Second statement**

*Salmosan* is classed as a POM-V

15 **First statement**

Magnesium phosphide is a part 1 schedule 1 poison

**Second statement**

Magnesium phosphide can be sold by a listed seller

16 **First statement**

Dangerous substances must be labelled with the appropriate safety phrases

**Second statement**

'Keep locked up' is a safety phrase detailed in the Approved Classification and Labelling Guide

17 **First statement**

A master of a ship can supply *Bach Rescue* cream to persons on the ship

**Second statement**

*Bach Rescue* cream is a general sales list medicine

18 **First statement**

Chiropodists can buy *Andrews Liver Salts* as wholesale from a pharmacy

**Second statement**

*Andrews Liver Salts* is a pharmacy-only medicine

19 **First statement**

Oil of croton must be sold in a fluted bottle

**Second statement**

This is a requirement made by the Medicines Regulations 1978 for this product

20 **First statement**

Midazolam is the only schedule 3 controlled drug that can be included in a patient group direction

**Second statement**

Under no other circumstances can controlled drugs be included in a patient group direction

21 **First statement**

It is a legal requirement for a detailed audit to be carried out by every person entitled to supply veterinary medicinal products at least once a year

**Second statement**

It is a legal requirement to audit stocks of authorised veterinary medicine – general sales list medicines

22 **First statement**

Surgical spirit is an industrial denatured alcohol

**Second statement**

There is no restriction on the quantity of surgical spirit that can be sold from a pharmacy

23 **First statement**

Safe custody applies to *all* controlled drugs

**Second statement**

Methylphenidate in an oral liquid form is exempt from safe custody

24 **First statement**

Co-fluampicil should not be given to patients with penicillin hypersensitivity

**Second statement**

Co-fluampicil is a broad-spectrum penicillin

25 **First statement**

Flucloxacillin should not be used in patients with a history of hepatic dysfunction

**Second statement**

Flucloxacillin may cause cholestatic jaundice

26 **First statement**

Quinolones may cause tendon damage

**Second statement**

Quinolones should not be given to patients with a history of quinolone sensitivity

27 **First statement**

Interferon gamma-1b should be used with caution in patients with seizure disorders

**Second statement**

Headache is a side-effect of this drug

28 **First statement**

*Prempak-C* levies 2 NHS prescription charges

**Second statement**

There are two different drugs and tablets contained within the calendar pack. *Prempak-C* contains 28 conjugated oestrogens and 12 norgestrel tablets

29 **First statement**

Triamcinolone is a corticosteroid

**Second statement**

10 mg prednisolone is equivalent to 8 mg triamcinolone (anti-inflammatory doses)

30 **First statement**

Doripenem is indicated for hospital-acquired pneumonia

**Second statement**

Antibiotic-associated colitis is a side-effect of doripenem

31 **First statement**

A maculopapular rash is commonly associated with ampicillin therapy

**Second statement**

A maculopapular rash is common in patients with glandular fever

32 **First statement**

Treatment with piroxicam gel should be reviewed 2 weeks after initiation

**Second statement**

There is an increased risk of serious skin reactions associated with the use of oral piroxicam

33 **First statement**

An angiotensin converting enzyme inhibitor may be the treatment of choice for younger Caucasians with hypertension.

**Second statement**

Renal disease is a possible cause of hypertension.

34 This question concerns the duties of the responsible pharmacist:

**First statement**

The responsible pharmacist is required to establish, maintain and review (at least once a year) the pharmacy procedures

**Second statement**

Examples of information that must be included in the procedures include circumstances where a pharmacy member may give medicinal advice and the record-keeping of this activity

35  This question concerns internet pharmacy services:

**First statement**

An online pharmacy must contain details on how to make a complaint about the pharmacy services

**Second statement**

The record-keeping of online consultations must include the information used for making the decision to supply the medicinal product

*The answers for this section are on pp. 74–76.*

## Open book answers

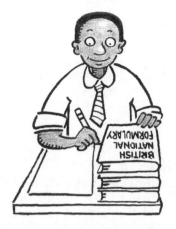

**1 A**
Tibolone is to be avoided in pregnancy. See BNF, Chapter 6 (Endocrine system), section 6.4.1.1, Oestrogens and HRT.

**2 D**
Acetylsalicylic acid (aspirin) should be avoided in severe hepatic impairment. See BNF, Chapter 4 (Central nervous system), section 4.7.1, Non-opioid analgesics.

**3 B**
Methysergide should be avoided in renal impairment. See BNF, Chapter 4 (Central nervous system), section 4.7.4.2, Prophylaxis of migraine.

**4 C**
See BNF, Appendix 1, Interactions.

**5 B**

**6 A**

**7 C**
See BNF, Appendix 1, Interactions.

**8 C**
See BNF, Appendix 6, Intravenous additives.

**9 D**
See BNF, Chapter 5 (Infections), section 5.1.4, Aminoglycosides; BNF, Appendix 6, Intravenous additives.

**10 B**
See BNF, Appendix 7.4, Feed supplements.

**11 E**
See BNF, Appendix 7.2, Nutritional supplements (non-disease-specific).

**12 C**
See BNF, Chapter 6 (Endocrine system), section 6.4.1.1, Oestrogens and HRT.

**13 C**
Abciximab should be used with caution in severe renal impairment. See BNF, Chapter 2 (Cardiovascular system), section 2.9, Antiplatelet drugs.

**14 A**
Methysergide should be avoided in hepatic impairment. See BNF, Chapter 4 (Central nervous system), section 4.7.4.2, Prophylaxis of migraine.

**15 B**
Tinzaparin should be avoided in breast-feeding. See BNF, Chapter 2 (Cardiovascular system), section 2.8.1, Parenteral anticoagulants.

**16 D**
Intrauterine progesterone-only system is not known to be harmful whilst breast-feeding. See BNF, Chapter 7 (Obstetrics, gynaecology, and urinary-tract disorders), section 7.3.2.3, Intrauterine progestogen-only device.

**17 B**
Thalidomide is known to be teratogenic. See BNF, Chapter 8 (Malignant disease and immunosuppression), section 8.2.4, Other immunomodulating drugs.

**18 C**
See BNF, Appendix 1, Interactions.

**19 D**
*Intrinsa* is monitored intensively by the MHRA. Drugs with a ▼ symbol are monitored intensively by the MHRA.

**20 B**
See BNF, Appendix 9, Cautionary and advisory labels for dispensed medicines.

**21 C**
See BNF, Appendix 9, Cautionary and advisory labels for dispensed medicines.

**22 D**
Piperacillin with tazobactam has the trade name *Tazocin*.

**23 E**
See BNF, Adverse reactions to drugs, Side-effects, and relevant drug monograph.

**24 D**
Calcium salts reduce the absorption of bisphosphonates and should not be taken on the same day. See BNF, Appendix 1, Interactions, List of drug interactions, Bisphosphonates.

**25 D**
*Clostridium difficile* is a Gram-positive anaerobe which produces a toxin that causes diarrhoea. This is a serious complication associated with some antibiotics such as amoxicillin, ciprofloxacin and clindamycin. It can be treated with oral metronidazole or vancomycin. *Salmonella, Shigella, Pseudomonas* and *Neisseria* are all Gram-negative bacteria. See BNF, Chapter 5 (Infections), Infections.

**26 D**
Polydipsia is normally associated with hyperglycaemia. See BNF, Guidance on prescribing, Prescribing in dental practice, Medical emergencies in dental practice, Hypoglycaemia.

**27 E**
*Bricanyl Turbohaler* contains terbutaline sulphate, which is a short-acting beta$_2$ agonist. All of these side-effects are common to beta$_2$ agonists, with the exception of arthralgia. Arthralgia is associated with salmeterol and not with terbutaline sulphate. See BNF, Chapter 3 (Respiratory system), section 3.1.1.1, Selective beta$_2$ agonists.

**28 C**
Low sodium is normally indicated by a sodium content of less than 1 mmol per tablet or 10 mL dose of a liquid preparation. Aromatic magnesium carbonate oral suspension contains 6 mmol of $Na^+$ per 10 mL dose. See BNF, Chapter 1 (Gastro-intestinal system), section 1.1.1, Antacids and simeticone.

**29 E**
Oestrogen-only products are suitable for use in women who have had a hysterectomy and do not suffer from endometriosis. *Zumenon* is the only preparation mentioned that consists of only an oestrogen (oestradiol); the others are combination preparations containing an oestrogen and a progestogen. See BNF, Chapter 6 (Endocrine system), section 6.4.1.1, Oestrogens and HRT, Hormone replacement therapy, Choice; Oestrogens for HRT, Conjugated oestrogens with progestogen; and Oestrogens for HRT, Estradiol only.

**30 C**
*Neocate Active* is powdered feed which is used as a dietary supplement in specific bowel conditions. See *Drug Tariff*, Appliances IXA/IXR and Borderline substances List A Part XV.

**31 C**
Only those appliances which are listed in Part IXA of the *Drug Tariff* are allowed to be prescribed on the NHS. *Bug Buster* kit can be found in *Drug Tariff* Part IXA, Head lice device.

**32 D**
*Bard Biocath* hydrogel coated Foley catheter does not have the heart symbol next to its name in Part IXA, Catheters, urinary, urethral of the *Drug Tariff* and therefore attracts a home delivery fee of £3.40.

**33 D**
See *Drug Tariff*, Part XV, Borderline substances, List B, Glycogen storage disease.

**34 D**
Community practitioner nurse prescriber can prescribe the listed products in *Drug Tariff*, Parts XVIIBi, IXA, IXB, IXC and IXR except where the ⃠ symbol appears.

**35 D**
Raloxifene 60 mg tablets is a category C drug hence the pharmacy will be reimbursed for the listed brand equivalent, *Evista*. See *Drug Tariff*, Part VIII, Basic prices of drugs.

**36 C**
See *Drug Tariff*, Part XVI, Notes on charges.

**37 D**
See *Drug Tariff*, Part XVI, Notes on charges.

**38 D**
See *Drug Tariff*, Part XVI, Notes on charges.

**39 E**
Any special item or sealed pack (in Part IX of the *Drug Tariff*) should not be opened (split/broken) during the dispensing process. See *Drug Tariff*, Part VIII, Basic price of drugs and Part IX, Appliances).

**40 E**
If the drug is not listed in Part VIII, Basic prices of drugs of the *Drug Tariff*, contractors should endorse the pack size and brand name (or manufacturer's/ wholesaler's name) of the drug. See *Drug Tariff*, Clause 9, Endorsement requirements.

**41 E**
Broken bulk can be claimed on drugs in categories A–C and M listed in Part VIII, Basic prices of drugs of the *Drug Tariff*. However broken bulk may be paid on ingredients of drugs in category E of Part VIII, Basic prices of drugs of the *Drug Tariff*.

**42 C**
*Delph* sun lotion SPF30 is not blacklisted. See *Drug Tariff*, Part XV, Borderline substances, List A; *Microalbustix* strips are not listed in Part IXR, Chemical reagents. The remaining items are all blacklisted; see Part XVIIIA.

**43 A**
*Clever Chek* strips are listed in Part IXR of the *Drug Tariff*, therefore can be supplied on the NHS.

**44 C**
This prescription should be referenced with 'SLS'. See *Drug Tariff*, Part XVIIIB.

**45 D**
Ponceau 4R (E124) is a red synthetic dye found in food, e.g. jelly. See inside back cover of the BNF, E numbers.

**46  C**
Avoid using dacarbazine as it has shown carcinogenicity and teratogenicity in animal studies. Men or woman taking this drug must use effective contraception during and for at least 6 months after treatment. See individual BNF entries.

**47  D**
Cimetidine can be sold to the public for adults and children over 16 years (provided packs do not contain more than 2 weeks' supply) for the short-term symptomatic relief of heartburn, dyspepsia and hyperacidity (maximum single dose 200 mg, maximum daily dose 800 mg), and for the prophylactic management of nocturnal heartburn (single nighttime dose 100 mg). See BNF, Chapter 1 (Gastro-intestinal system), section 1.3.1, H$_2$-receptor antagonists, Cimetidine.

**48  E**
The question is referring to an established drug, thus only serious reactions such as fatal, life-threatening, disabling or incapacitating reactions should be reported to the MHRA regardless of whether or not they are a recognised or a new effect. This includes effects on fertility. See BNF, Chapter 2 (Cardiovascular system), section 2.2.1, Thiazides and related diuretics; and Guidance on prescribing, Adverse reactions to drugs.

**49  C**
See BNF, Chapter 9 (Nutrition and blood), section 9.1.5, G6PD deficiency.

**50  E**
*Zimovane* is the brand name for the hypnotic zopiclone. See individual BNF drug entries.

**51  C**
Excessive daytime sleepiness and sudden onset of sleep can occur with co-careldopa, co-beneldopa and dopamine receptor agonists, e.g. pramipexole (*Mirapexin*). Mrs J should also be advised not to drive until these effects have stopped occurring. See BNF, Chapter 4 (Central nervous system), section 4.9.1, Dopaminergic drugs used in parkinsonism.

**52  D**
See BNF, Chapter 10 (Musculoskeletal and joint diseases), section 10.1.1, Non-steroidal anti-inflammatory drugs, Tiaprofenic acid, CSM advice.

**53 D**
See BNF, Chapter 1 (Gastro-intestinal system), section 1.1.1, Antacids and simeticone; section 1.1.2, Compound alginates and proprietary indigestion preparations, Other compound alginate preparations.

**54 E**
Nandrolone is an anabolic steroid. This class of drugs is listed in BNF, Chapter 9 (Nutrition and blood), section 9.8.2, Acute porphyrias, Drugs unsafe for use in acute porphyrias of the BNF.

**55 C**
See individual BNF entries, Renal impairment.

**56 E**
See BNF, Chapter 13 (Skin), section 13.4, Topical corticosteroids, Clobetasol propionate, *Etrivex*.

**57 C**
See BNF, Chapter 2 (Cardiovascular system), section 2.12, Lipid-regulating drugs, Statins, Side-effects of pravastatin sodium.

**58 C**
SSRIs are better tolerated and are safer in overdose than other classes of antidepressants and should be considered first-line treatment for depression. See BNF, Chapter 4 (Central nervous system), section 4.3.4, Other antidepressant drugs.

**59 D**
Extrapyramidal symptoms occur most frequently with the piperazine phenothiazines (fluphenazine, perphenazine, prochlorperazine and trifluoperazine), the butyrophenones (benperidol and haloperidol) and the depot preparations. See BNF, Chapter 4 (Central nervous system), section 4.2.1, Antipsychotic drugs, Side-effects.

**60 E**
See BNF, Emergency treatment of poisoning, Specific drugs, Iron salts.

**61 C**
See BNF, Appendix 1, Interactions, List of drug interactions, Barbiturates.

**62 D**
*Remedeine* tablets contain paracetamol and dihydrocodeine. Note that aspirin and other NSAIDs are contraindicated in individuals who are hypersensitive or have shown hypersensitivity (e.g. asthma attack, angioedema, urticaria or rhinitis) to either aspirin or any other NSAIDs. See BNF, Chapter 4 (Central nervous system), section 4.7.1, Non-opioid analgesics, Aspirin.

**63 C**
See BNF, Chapter 9 (Nutrition and blood), section 9.2.1.2, Oral sodium and water, Oral rehydration therapy (ORT).

**64 B**
See BNF, Chapter 3 (Respiratory system), section 2.5.5.2, Angiotensin-II receptor antagonists, *Amias*; 2 mg (white), 4 mg (white and scored) and 8 mg, 16 mg or 32 mg (pink and scored).

**65 C**
Dicycloverine hydrochloride is POM but P if maximum single dose (MD) is 10 mg and maximum daily dose (MDD) is 60 mg. See MEP, Section 1.3, Alphabetical list of medicines for human use, Dicycloverine hydrochloride.

**66 E**
All are listed except acetylcysteine. See MEP, Section 1.2.3, Prescription-only medicines (POM), Administration of parenteral medicines for the purpose of saving a life in an emergency.

**67 A**
See MEP, Section 1.2.6.8, Labelling of products for pharmacy sale only, part (7).

**68 E**
See MEP, Section 1.2.4, Wholesale dealing, Recording of wholesale supplies of prescription-only medicines.

**69 E**
Benzfetamine is CD no reg. See MEP, Section 1.2.14, Controlled drugs, Prescriptions for controlled drugs; Section 1.3, Alphabetical list of medicines for human use.

**70 D**
See MEP, Section 1.2.14, Controlled drugs, Obsolete, expired and unwanted stock controlled drugs; or Methods and procedures, Alphabetical list of medicines for human use.

**71 E**
Emergency supplies at the request of a patient can be made for phenobarbital and controlled drugs in schedules 4 (both parts) and 5. See MEP, Section 1.2.3, Prescription-only medicines (POM), Emergency supplies of prescription-only medicines, Supply made at the request of a patient.

**72 A**
See MEP, Section 1.2.6.1, Labelling of dispensed relevant medicinal products.

**73 E**
A pharmacist is allowed to disclose confidential information about patients without their consent only to specific persons under specific circumstances. This includes disclosure of information to a police officer (or NHS fraud investigating officer) only if he or she provides written confirmation that the disclosure is necessary to assist in the prevention, detection or prosecution of serious crime. See MEP, Section 2.2, Professional standards and guidance documents for patient confidentiality, Releasing information without consent.

## MULTIPLE COMPLETION ANSWERS

**1 A**

All three are side-effects. See BNF, Chapter 5 (Infections), section 5.2.1, Triazole antifungals.

**2 A**

All three are safe to give in pregnancy. See under each individual drug in the BNF.

**3 B**

Bleomycin and doxorubicin are used in the treatment of non-Hodgkin's lymphoma. See BNF, Chapter 8 (Malignant disease and immunosuppression), section 8.1.2, Anthracyclines and other cytotoxic antibiotics.

**4 C**

Ganirelix and alendronic acid are to be avoided in moderate renal failure. See under each drug in the BNF for a full explanation.

**5 E**

Disulfiram is indicated for the treatment of alcohol dependence. See BNF, Chapter 4 (Central nervous system), section 4.10, Drugs used in substance dependence.

**6 B**

See BNF, Chapter 4 (Central nervous system), section 4.7.4.1, Treatment of acute migraine.

**7 D**

Pyridoxine is used for the treatment of vitamin $B_6$ deficiency. See BNF, Chapter 9 (Nutrition and blood), section 9.6.2, Vitamin B group.

**8 A**

All three have a definite risk of haemolysis in G6PD-deficient individuals. See BNF, Chapter 9 (Nutrition and blood), section 9.1.5, G6PD deficiency.

**9 C**

Quinine and probenecid have a possible risk of haemolysis in G6PD-deficient individuals. See BNF, Chapter 9 (Nutrition and blood), section 9.1.5, G6PD deficiency.

**10 D**
Pamaquin has a definite risk of haemolysis in G6PD-deficient individuals. See BNF, Chapter 9 (Nutrition and blood), section 9.1.5, G6PD deficiency.

**11 D**
MMR is cautioned in these individuals. However, influenza vaccine (prepared in hens' eggs), tick-borne encephalitis vaccine and yellow fever vaccine are all contraindicated in individuals with a history of an anaphylactic reaction to eggs. See BNF, Chapter 14 (Immunological products and vaccines), section 14.1, Active immunity, Contra-indications.

**12 D**
See *Drug Tariff*, Part IXA, Appliances, Elastic hosiery.

**13 E**
*Advagraf* is a prolonged-release preparation that is administered only once daily; the other two preparations are immediate-release preparations which are taken twice daily. See BNF, Chapter 8 (Malignant disease and immunosuppression), section 8.2.2, Corticosteroids and other immunosuppressants, Tacrolimus.

**14 A**
Some cases of male breast cancer have been reported with finasteride, therefore patients or their carers should be advised to report any changes in their breast tissue (e.g. lumps, pain or discharge) to their doctors immediately. See BNF, Chapter 6 (Endocrine system), section 6.4.2, Male sex hormones and antagonists, Anti-androgens, Dutasteride and finasteride.

Carbimazole may induce bone marrow suppression. Patients who take carbimazole and develop a sore throat (or any other sign of infection) must stop treatment and seek medical attention immediately. See BNF, Chapter 6 (Endocrine system), section 6.2.2, Antithyroid drugs, Carbimazole.

Patients who are taking tiaprofenic acid should be advised to stop treatment and seek medical attention if they develop urinary tract symptoms such as increased frequency, urgency, nocturia, pain on urinating or blood in urine. See BNF, Chapter 10 (Musculoskeletal and joint diseases), section 10.1.1, Non-steroidal anti-inflammatory drugs, Tiaprofenic acid.

**15 D**
See BNF, Guidance on prescribing, General guidance, Excipients.

**16 E**
Xerostomia is the medical term used to describe dry mouth and is associated with drugs that exhibit antimuscarinic side-effects such as hyoscine and clozapine. See corresponding drug monographs.

**17 D**
See BNF, Chapter 5 (Infections), section 5.4.1, Antimalarials, Pregnancy.

**18 B**
See BNF, Chapter 13 (Skin), section 13.10.4, Parasiticidal preparations.

**19 B**
See BNF, Chapter 11 (Eye), section 11.8.1, Tear deficiency, ocular lubricants, and astringents, Carbomers.

**20 D**
See MEP, Section 1.2.2, Pharmacy medicines, Responsible pharmacist.

**21 A**
Naproxen 250 mg is licensed for the treatment of primary dysmenorrhoea in women between the ages of 15 and 50 but for a maximum of 3 days' treatment. See MEP, Section 1.3, Alphabetical list of medicines for human use: refer to separate entries.

**22 E**
See MEP, Section 1.2.8, Use of fluted bottles.

**23 A**
See MEP, Section 1.7.4, Conditions of use of IDA and TSDA, Distribution.

**24 D**
See MEP, Section 1.8.3, Records.

**25 B**
See MEP, Section 1.8.1, Prescriptions, Controlled drug prescription, and Section 1.8.3, Records.

**26 C**
The Suspected Adverse Reaction Surveillance Scheme monitors and records adverse reactions to veterinary or human medicines in both animals and humans. See MEP, Section 1.8.11, Suspected adverse reactions.

**27 E**
Prescribers who request an emergency supply have 72 hours in which to issue a prescription. See MEP, Section 1.2.3, Prescription-only medicines (POM), Emergency supplies of prescription-only medicines.

**28 C**
See MEP, Section 1.2.4, Wholesale dealing.

**29 B**
See MEP, Section 1.6.1, Supply requirements.

**30 E**
See MEP, Section 1.2.14, Controlled drugs, National Health prescriptions for the treatment of misusers; Private controlled drug prescriptions; Prescriptions for controlled drugs.

**31 E**
See MEP, Section 1.2.14, Controlled drugs, Requisitions for schedule 1, 2 and 3 controlled drugs; Supply of controlled drugs from the community.

**32 B**
See MEP, Section 1.2.14, Controlled drugs, Technical errors on controlled drug prescriptions; Destruction of controlled drugs, Patient-returned controlled drugs and Authorised witness.

**33 B**
See MEP, Section 1.2.1, General sale list medicines (GSL), Pharmacy only (PO); Section 1.2.2, Pharmacy medicines (P), Responsible pharmacist; Section 1.2.3, Prescription-only medicines (POM), Exemptions to medicines legislation in the event of a pandemic.

**34 C**
*Lanoxin* injection is given intermittently in glucose 5% or sodium chloride 0.9% over 2 hours and must be protected from exposure to the light. See BNF, Chapter 2 (Cardiovascular system), section 2.1.1, Cardiac glycosides, Digoxin and Appendix 6, Intravenous additives, Digoxin.

**35 C**
Statement 1 is incorrect because containers for short-acting tablets must not contain cotton wool wadding. See BNF, Chapter 2 (Cardiovascular system), section 2.6.1, Nitrates, Glyceryl trinitrate.

**36 D**
Patients or their carers can report suspected adverse reactions to the MHRA via the Yellow Card scheme. The symbol ▼ represents newly licensed medicines. Any adverse effects from these medicines should be reported to the MHRA, even those thought to be less significant. See BNF, Guidance on prescribing, Adverse reactions to drugs.

**37 C**
Carbimazole may induce bone marrow suppression; patients must therefore report any signs of infection or bruising immediately. See BNF, Chapter 6 (Endocrine system), section 6.2.2, Antithyroid drugs, CSM warning, Neutropenia and agranulocytosis.

**38 B**
See BNF, Chapter 4 (Central nervous system), section 4.8.1, Control of epilepsy, Gabapentin.

**39 A**
Miss E should also be advised to see her doctor for contraceptive medication as isotretinoin is teratogenic and patients taking it should practise effective contraceptive measures 1 month before, during and for 1 month after treatment. Note that progestogen-only contraceptives may not be effective. See BNF, Chapter 13 (Skin), section 13.6.2, Oral preparations for acne, Oral retinoid for acne, Isotretinoin, Pregnancy prevention/counselling.

**40 A**
See BNF, Chapter 5 (Infections), section 5, Infections, Notifiable diseases.

**41 E**
See BNF, Chapter 5 (Infections), section 5, Infections, Table 1, Summary of antibacterial treatment, Respiratory system.

**42 A**
All contain iodine. See individual BNF entries.

**43 B**
Any adverse reactions (including minor reactions) in children under the age of 18 years should be reported to the MHRA immediately. See BNF, Guidance on prescribing, Adverse reactions to drugs and Yellow Card scheme.

**44 D**
Dosage adjustments must be made for patients at both weight extremes (BMI $<18.5\,kg/m^2$ or $>30\,kg/m^2$) and the serum creatinine levels can only be used as a rough guide to dosing. See BNF, Guidance on prescribing, Prescribing in renal impairment, Principles of dose adjustment in renal impairment.

**45 C**
Statement 1 is incorrect because doses of intramuscular injections should ideally be lower than their corresponding oral dosages owing to absence of the first-pass effect in IM injections. This is especially important in very active individuals, who have an increased blood flow to their muscles and a higher rate of drug absorption. See BNF, Chapter 4 (Central nervous system), section 4.2, Drugs used in psychoses and related disorders.

**46 E**
Advice should be obtained from the National Poisons Information Service on the management of hypertension caused by amphetamine use. See BNF, Guidance on prescribing, Emergency treatment of poisoning, Specific drugs, Stimulants, Amphetamines.

**47 B**
The manufacturer advises to dispense *Asasantin Retard* in its original container (it contains a desiccant) and to discard any remaining capsules 6 weeks after opening. Labels 21 and 25 apply to *Asasantin Retard*. See BNF, Chapter 2 (Cardiovascular system), section 2.9, Antiplatelet drugs, *Asasantin Retard* and Recommended wording of cautionary and advisory labels.

**48 A**
Some oily products, including petroleum jelly, baby oil and oil-based vaginal and rectal preparations, are likely to damage condoms and contraceptive diaphragms made from latex rubber, and may render them less effective as a barrier method of contraception and as protection from sexually transmitted diseases such as HIV. See BNF, Chapter 7 (Obstetrics, gynaecology, and urinary-tract disorders), section 7.3.3, Spermicidal contraceptives.

**49 B**
Carmellose Gelatin Paste DPF is listed as a medical device under Oral film forming agents, *Orabase* paste in Part IXA of the *Drug Tariff*. Saliva *Orthana* is listed in Part XVIIA, Dental prescribing under artificial saliva and can be prescribed on FP10D forms only for indications which are approved by the ACBS.

**50  A**
See *Drug Tariff*, Part IXA, Appliances, Contraceptive devices, Vaginal contraceptive caps (pessaries) and Part XVI, Notes on charges, Contraceptive services. Also see BNF, Chapter 7 (Obstetrics, gynaecology, and urinary-tract disorders), section 7.3.3, Spermicidal contraceptives.

**51  D**
Category E products automatically attract the relevant additional fee listed in *Drug Tariff*, Part IIIA 2A. Only drugs in schedules 2 and 3 attract the specified additional fee. See *Drug Tariff*, Part IIIA, Professional fees and Part VIII, Basic prices of drugs.

**52  D**
Pharmacists/contractors should endorse NHS prescriptions containing specials with 'DNG' to avoid discount being removed. This is not necessary for items already listed in Part II, Drugs for which discount is not deducted, of the latest *Drug Tariff*.

**53  E**
Only doxycycline 100 mg capsules or doxycycline 20 mg tablets DPF can be prescribed on an NHS dentist prescription. See *Drug Tariff*, Part XVIIA, Dental prescribing.

**54  C**
See *Drug Tariff*, Part II, Clause 12, Out of pocket expenses.

**55  C**
Two puffs of the *Respimat* solution are equivalent to 5 micrograms of tiotropium. See BNF, Chapter 3 (Respiratory system), section 3.1.2, Antimuscarinic bronchodilators, Tiotropium, *Spiriva*.

**56  E**
5 mg prednisolone is equivalent to 20 mg hydrocortisone, with respect to anti-inflammatory activity. Prednisolone has more glucocorticoid activity than hydrocortisone and its side-effects include diabetes and osteoporosis. See BNF, Chapter 6 (Endocrine system), section 6.3.2, Glucocorticoid therapy, Equivalent anti-inflammatory doses of corticosteroids, Prednisolone, and Side-effects of corticosteroids, Glucocorticoid.

**57 D**

The dose of antidepressant drugs should be reduced over 4 or more weeks prior to stopping therapy. See BNF, Chapter 4 (Central nervous system), section 4.3, Antidepressant drugs, Choice, and Withdrawal.

**58 A**

See relevant drug monographs in the BNF.

**59 D**

Statement 1 is correct. See BNF, Chapter 11 (Eye), section 11.8.2, Ocular diagnostic and peri-operative preparations, and photodynamic treatment, Ocular diagnostic preparations. *Diabur-Test 5000* is used to detect glucose in urine. See BNF, Chapter 6 (Endocrine system), section 6.1.6, Diagnostic and monitoring devices for diabetes mellitus, Urinalysis. A patient is diagnosed with adrenal insufficiency when the plasma cortisol concentration fails to rise following administration of tetracosactide. See BNF, Chapter 6 (Endocrine system), section 6.5.1, Hypothalamic and anterior pituitary hormones and anti-oestrogens, Anterior pituitary hormones, Corticotrophins.

## CLASSIFICATION ANSWERS

**1 D**
See BNF, Chapter 11 (Eye), section 11.6, Treatment of glaucoma.

**2 B**
See BNF, Chapter 4 (Central nervous system), section 4.7.4.2, Prophylaxis of migraine.

**3 A**
See BNF, Chapter 4 (Central nervous system), section 4.6, Drugs used in nausea and vertigo.

**4 C**
See BNF, Chapter 10 (Musculoskeletal and joint diseases), section 10.1.1, Non-steroidal anti-inflammatory drugs.

**5 B**
See BNF, Chapter 4 (Central nervous system), section 4.7.4.2, Prophylaxis of migraine.

**6 E**
See BNF, Chapter 8 (Malignant disease and immunosuppression), section 8.3.4.2, Gonadorelin analogues and gonadotrophin-releasing hormone antagonists.

**7 C**
See BNF, Chapter 6 (Endocrine system), section 6.7.2, Drugs affecting gonadotrophins.

**8 C**
See BNF, Chapter 6 (Endocrine system), section 6.7.2, Drugs affecting gonadotrophins.

**9 B**
See BNF, Chapter 5 (Infections), section 5.3.2.1, Herpes simplex and varicella-zoster infection.

**10 A**
See BNF, Chapter 5 (Infections), section 5.1.7, Some other antibacterials.

**11 E**
See BNF, Chapter 1 (Gastro-intestinal system), section 1.6.7, $5HT_4$ receptor agonists.

**12 A**
See BNF, Chapter 6 (Endocrine system), section 6.4.1.1, Oestrogens and HRT.

**13 B**
See BNF, Chapter 10 (Musculoskeletal and joint diseases), section 10.1.1, Non-steroidal anti-inflammatory drugs.

**14 C**
See BNF, Chapter 13 (Skin), section 13.2.2, Barrier preparations.

**15 D**
See BNF, Chapter 4 (Central nervous system), section 4.1.1, Hypnotics.

**16 D**
See BNF, Chapter 4 (Central nervous system), section 4.1.1, Hypnotics.

**17 E**
See BNF, Chapter 1 (Gastro-intestinal system), section 1.6.7, $5HT_4$ receptor agonists.

**18 A**
See BNF, Chapter 6 (Endocrine system), section 6.4.1.1, Oestrogens and HRT.

**19 B**
See BNF, Chapter 10 (Musculoskeletal and joint diseases), section 10.1.1, Non-steroidal anti-inflammatory drugs.

**20 C**
See BNF, Chapter 13 (Skin), section 13.2.2, Barrier preparations.

**21 E**
See BNF, Chapter 2 (Cardiovascular system), section 2.8.2, Oral anticoagulants.

**22 E**
See BNF, Chapter 2 (Cardiovascular system), section 2.8.2, Oral anticoagulants.

**23 B**
See BNF, Chapter 6 (Endocrine system), section 6.2.2, Antithyroid drugs.

**24 A**
See BNF, Chapter 5 (Infections), section 5.1.9, Antituberculosis drugs.

**25 C**
See BNF, Chapter 3 (Respiratory system), section 3.1.5, Peak flow meters, inhaler devices and nebulisers.

**26 D**
See BNF, Chapter 2 (Cardiovascular system), section 2.9, Antiplatelet drugs.

**27 E**
See BNF, Chapter 2 (Cardiovascular system), section 2.8.2, Oral anticoagulants.

**28 C**
See BNF, Chapter 3 (Respiratory system), section 3.1.5, Peak flow meters, inhaler devices and nebulisers.

**29 B**
See BNF, Chapter 6 (Endocrine system), section 6.2.2, Antithyroid drugs.

**30 A**
See BNF, Chapter 5 (Infections), section 5.1.9, Antituberculosis drugs.

**31 D**
See BNF, Chapter 2 (Cardiovascular system), section 2.12, Lipid-regulating drugs.

**32 C**
See BNF, Chapter 2 (Cardiovascular system), section 2.6.2, Calcium-channel blockers.

**33 B**
See BNF, Chapter 2 (Cardiovascular system), section 2.4, Beta-adrenoceptor blocking drugs.

**34 A**
See BNF, Chapter 2 (Cardiovascular system), section 2.5.5, Drugs affecting the renin–angiotensin system.

**35 E**
See BNF, Chapter 4 (Central nervous system), section 4.8.1, Control of epilepsy.

**36 B**
See BNF, Chapter 2 (Cardiovascular system), section 2.4, Beta-adrenoceptor blocking drugs.

**37 B**
See BNF, Chapter 2 (Cardiovascular system), section 2.4, Beta-adrenoceptor blocking drugs.

**38 A**
See BNF, Chapter 2 (Cardiovascular system), section 2.5.5, Drugs affecting the renin–angiotensin system.

**39 E**
See BNF, Chapter 4 (Central nervous system), section 4.8.1, Control of epiliepsy.

**40 C**
See BNF, Chapter 2 (Cardiovascular system), section 2.6.2, Calcium-channel blockers.

**41 A**
See BNF, Chapter 4 (Central nervous system), section 4.1.1, Hypnotics.

**42 B**
See BNF, Chapter 4 (Central nervous system), section 4.8.1, Control of epilepsy.

**43 C**
See BNF, Chapter 6 (Endocrine system), section 6.6.1, Calcitonin and parathyroid hormone.

**44 C**
See BNF, Chapter 6 (Endocrine system), section 6.6.1, Calcitonin and parathyroid hormone.

**45 D**
See BNF, Chapter 8 (Malignant disease and immunosuppression), section 8.1.5, Other antineoplastic drugs.

**46 D**
See BNF, Chapter 8 (Malignant disease and immunosuppression), section 8.1.5, Other antineoplastic drugs.

**47 E**
See BNF, Chapter 2 (Cardiovascular system), section 2.3.2, Drugs for arrhythmias.

**48 E**
See BNF, Chapter 2 (Cardiovascular system), section 2.3.2, Drugs for arrhythmias.

**49 A**
See BNF, Chapter 4 (Central nervous system), section 4.1.1, Hypnotics.

**50 B**
See BNF, Chapter 4 (Central nervous system), section 4.8.1, Control of epilepsy.

**51 D**
See BNF, Chapter 2 (Cardiovascular system), section 2.8.1, Parenteral anticoagulants.

**52 C**
See BNF, Chapter 2 (Cardiovascular system), section 2.9, Antiplatelet drugs.

**53 B**
See BNF, Chapter 3 (Respiratory system), section 3.7, Mucolytics.

**54 A**
See BNF, Chapter 4 (Central nervous system), section 4.2.1, Antipsychotic drugs.

**55 A**
See BNF, Chapter 4 (Central nervous system), section 4.2.1, Antipsychotic drugs.

**56 A**
See BNF, Chapter 4 (Central nervous system), section 4.2.1, Antipsychotic drugs.

**57 E**
See BNF, Chapter 2 (Cardiovascular system), section 2.5.2, Centrally acting antihypertensive drugs.

**58 E**
See BNF, Chapter 2 (Cardiovascular system), section 2.5.1, Vasodilator antihypertensive drugs.

**59 D**
See BNF, Chapter 2 (Cardiovascular system), section 2.8.1, Parenteral anticoagulants.

**60 B**
See BNF, Chapter 3 (Respiratory system), section 3.7, Mucolytics.

**61 A**
See BNF, Chapter 2 (Cardiovascular system), section 2.2.3, Potassium-sparing diuretics and aldosterone antagonists, Amiloride hydrochloride.

**62 D**
See BNF, Appendix 1, Interactions, List of drug interactions, Thyroid hormones.

**63 D**
See BNF, Chapter 9 (Nutrition and blood), section 9.5, Minerals.

**64 B**
See BNF, Chapter 9 (Nutrition and blood), section 9.5.1.3, Magnesium.

**65 D**
See BNF, Chapter 9 (Nutrition and blood), section 9.5.2, Phosphorus.

**66 A**
Clenbuterol is CD Anab POM. See MEP, Section 1.3, Alphabetical list of medicines for human use for classification of CD schedules, and Schedule 4 drugs (CD Benz POM or CD Anab POM) monograph.

**67 C**
See MEP, Section 1.3, Alphabetical list of medicines for human use for classification of CD schedules: hexobarbitone and phenobarbital are CD No Reg but hexobarbitone is not exempt from safe custody as it is not listed under 'safe custody of controlled drugs' and phenobarbital is. Quinalbarbitone is the only CD POM which does not require safe custody. See Schedule 2 drugs (CD POM) monograph.

**68 C**
See MEP, Section 1.2.5, Sales of medicines to exempted organisations, healthcare professionals or other persons, Chiropodists' list for patient administration.

**69 D**
The restrictions on sale or supply of POMs, P medicines or GSLs do not apply to dentists or doctors when sold/supplied to their patients. See MEP, Section 1.2.5, Sales of medicines to exempted organisations, healthcare professionals or other persons, Practitioners; and *Drug Tariff*, Part XVIIB, Dental prescribing.

**70 B**
See MEP, Section 1.3, Alphabetical list of medicines for human use.

**71 D**
See MEP, Section 1.3, Alphabetical list of medicines for human use.

**72 D**
LSD is CD Lic. See MEP, Section 1.3, Alphabetical list of medicines for human use, for classification of CD schedules and related monograph.

**73 C**
*Codipar* caplets are CD POM Inv. See MEP, Section 1.3, Alphabetical list of medicines for human use, for classification of CD schedules and related monograph.

**74 A**
*Acumed* patch is GSL. *Mandanol* 32 tablets/*Cystofem*/*Nylax* with senna 30 tablets are PO products which can only be sold from registered pharmacies but don't have to be under the supervision of the pharmacist. See MEP, Section 1.3, Alphabetical list of medicines for human use.

**75 D**
*Daktarin* (Janssen-Cilag) oral gel is POM. See MEP, Section 1.3, Alphabetical list of medicines for human use.

**76 B**
The advisory label 'with plenty of water' is used for preparations where dilution is required (e.g. chioral hydrate such as *Welldorm* preparations), where a high fluid intake is required (e.g. sulphonamides) or where water is required to aid the action (e.g. methylcellulose). See BNF, Appendix 9, Cautionary and advisory labels for dispensed medicines, Recommended label wordings.

**77 E**
Penicillamine chelates calcium, iron and zinc, which are present in some indigestion products. This leads to poor drug absorption when taken at the same time. However, these incompatible preparations can be taken 2–3 hours apart. See BNF, Appendix 9, Cautionary and advisory labels for dispensed medicines, Recommended label wordings.

**78 D**
Preparations containing clioquinol will stain users' skin and clothes. See BNF, Chapter 12 (Ear, nose, and oropharynx), section 12.1.1, Otitis externa, Anti-infective preparations, *Locorten-Vioform*.

**79 C**
See BNF, Chapter 13 (Skin), section 13.4, Topical corticosteroids, Topical corticosteroid preparation potencies.

**80 B**
*Roaccutane* capsules may contain arachis (peanut) oil. See BNF, Chapter 13 (Skin), section 13.6.2, Oral preparations for acne, Isotretinoin, *Roaccutane*.

**81 E**
Cabergoline (brand or generic) should be dispensed in its original container as it contains a desiccant. See BNF, Chapter 6 (Endocrine system), section 6.7.1, Bromocriptine and other dopaminergic drugs, Cabergoline.

**82 A**
Minocycline tablets or capsules should be swallowed whole with plenty of fluid while sitting or standing. See BNF, Chapter 5 (Infections), section 5.1.3, Tetracyclines, Minocycline.

**83 D**
*Gygel* contains the excipients hydroxybenzoates (parabens), propylene glycol (E1520) and sorbic acid (E200). See BNF, Chapter 7 (Obstetrics, gynaecology, and urinary-tract disorders), section 7.3.3, Spermicidal contraceptives, *Gygel*, and E numbers on the inside back cover of the BNF.

**84 D**
See BNF, Chapter 4 (Central nervous system), section 4.2.1, Antipsychotic drugs, Risperidone, Orodispersible tablets.

**85 B**
See BNF, Chapter 1 (Gastro-intestinal system), section 1.3.5, Proton pump inhibitors, Omeprazole, *Losec, MUPS*.

**86 A**
Grapefruit juice increases the plasma concentration of ciclosporin, thus increasing the risk of toxicity. See BNF, Appendix 1, Interactions, List of drug interactions, Grapefruit juice.

**87 C**
Alcohol causes etretinate to be formed from acitretin. This increases the risk of teratogenecity in women of child-bearing potential. See BNF, Appendix 1, Interactions, List of drug interactions, Alcohol.

**88 B**
There have been reports of bezoar formation with sucralfate. The CSM has advised caution in seriously ill patients, especially those receiving concomitant enteral feeds or those with predisposing conditions such as delayed gastric emptying. See BNF, Chapter 1 (Gastro-intestinal system), section 1.3.3, Chelates and complexes, Sucralfate.

**89 D**
See BNF, Chapter 11 (Eye), section 11.4.1, Corticosteroids, Loteprednol etabonate.

**90 E**
See BNF, Appendix 9, Cautionary and advisory labels for dispensed medicines.

**91 A**
See BNF, Appendix 9, Cautionary and advisory labels for dispensed medicines.

**92 D**
See BNF, Chapter 3 (Respiratory system), section 3.3.1, Cromoglicate and related therapy, *Tilade* CFC-free inhaler.

**93 A**
See BNF, Chapter 2 (Cardiovascular system), section 2.5.5, Drugs affecting the renin–angiotensin system, Quinapril, *Accupro*.

**94 B**
See BNF, Appendix 9, Cautionary and advisory labels for dispensed medicines.

**95 C**
See BNF, Appendix 9, Cautionary and advisory labels for dispensed medicines.

## STATEMENT ANSWERS

**1 D**
See MEP, Section 1.2.14, Controlled drugs, Destruction of controlled drugs.

**2 B**
See MEP, Section 1.2.14, Controlled drugs, Controlled drugs and midwives.

**3 B**
See MEP, Section 1.2.14, Controlled drugs, Electronic controlled drug registers.

**4 D**
See MEP, Section 1.2.14, Controlled drugs, Collection of schedule 2 and 3 CDs.

**5 D**
See MEP, Section 1.2.14, Controlled drugs, Prescribing for up to 30 days' clinical need.

**6 B**
See MEP, Section 1.2.14, Controlled drugs, Schedule 1 drugs.

**7 A**
See MEP, Section 1.2.14, Controlled drugs, Secretary of State prohibitions.

**8 B**
See MEP, Section 1.2.11, Chloroform: sale and supply.

**9 A**
See MEP, Section 1.2.4, Wholesale dealing.

**10 B**
See MEP, Section 1.2.

**11 B**
See MEP, Section 1.2.13, Handling of waste medicines, Scotland.

**12 E**
See MEP, Section 1.2.10, Restrictions on the sale of plano cosmetic lenses. The Opticians Act was passed in 1989, not 1984.

**13 B**
See MEP, Section 1.7.1, Type of denatured alcohol.

**14 A**
See MEP, Sections 1.8 and 1.9, Medicines for veterinary use.

**15 C**
Part 1 poisons can only be supplied/sold by persons lawfully conducting retail pharmacy business.

**16 B**
See MEP, Section 1.6.2.1, Chemicals, Supply requirements, and Sections 1.4 and 1.5, Non-medicinal poisons.

**17 A**
See MEP, Section 1.2.5, Sales of medicines to exempted organisations, healthcare professionals or other persons.

**18 C**
See MEP, Section 1.2.5, Sales of medicines to exempted organisations, healthcare professionals or other persons.

**19 A**
See MEP, Section 1.2.8, Use of fluted bottles.

**20 C**
See MEP, Section 1.2.14, Controlled drugs and patient group directions.

**21 C**
See MEP, Section 1.8, Medicines for veterinary use.

**22 D**
See MEP, Section 1.7.4, Use of IDA and TSDA.

**23 D**
See MEP, Section 1.2.14, Controlled drugs.

**24 A**
See BNF, Chapter 5 (Infections), section 5.1.1.3, Broad-spectrum penicillins.

**25 A**
See BNF, Chapter 5 (Infections), section 5.1.1.2, Penicillinase-resistant penicillins.

**26 B**
See BNF, Chapter 5 (Infections), section 5.1.1.2, Penicillinase-resistant penicillins.

**27 B**
See BNF, Chapter 8 (Malignant disease and immunosuppression), section 8.2.4, Other immunomodulating drugs.

**28 A**
See BNF, Chapter 6 (Endocrine system), section 6.4.1, Female sex hormones.

**29 B**
See BNF, Chapter 6 (Endocrine system), section 6.3.2, Glucocorticoid therapy.

**30 B**
See BNF, Chapter 5 (Infections), section 5.1.2.2, Carbapenems.

**31 B**
See BNF, Chapter 5 (Infections), section 5.1.1.3, Broad-spectrum penicillins, Ampicillin.

**32 D**
Restrictions on the use of piroxicam only apply to the oral preparations, not the topical preparations. See BNF, Chapter 10 (Musculoskeletal and joint diseases), section 10.1.1, Non-steroidal anti-inflammatory drugs, Piroxicam, CHMP advice.

**33 B**
See BNF, Chapter 2 (Cardiovascular system), sections 2.5, Hypertension and heart failure, and 2.5.5.1, Angiotensin-converting enzyme inhibitors.

**34 D**
Pharmacy procedures can be reviewed once every 2 years See MEP 33, Section 2.2, Professional standards and guidance for responsible pharmacists and Appendix A.

**35 B**
The first statement outlines the display requirements for a pharmacy website whereas the second statement refers to the particulars to record for online consultations. See MEP 33, Section 2.2, Professional standards and guidance for internet pharmacy services, 2, Website requirements; and 9, Record keeping.

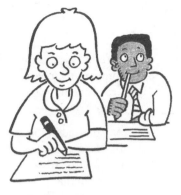

# Closed book questions

Nadia Bukhari and Naba Elsaid

## SIMPLE COMPLETION QUESTIONS

Each of the questions or statements in this section is followed by five suggested answers. Select the best answer in each situation.

1 Which of the following drugs should be initiated at bedtime?

    A   enalapril
    B   propranolol
    C   digoxin
    D   bendroflumethazide
    E   clopidogrel

2 Mr Chowdhury has been prescribed orlistat by his GP. What is the indication for this drug?

    A   major depressive disorder
    B   hyperlipidaemia
    C   tonic-clonic seizures
    D   adjunct in obesity
    E   fungal infection

3 Mrs Sisstanem is suffering with acute pain in her legs. Her pain started 2 weeks ago, for which she took regular paracetamol. The pain improved; however, over the past 2 days she has been feeling pain again in her legs. Her GP has recommended that she take a weak opioid in addition to the paracetamol. Which of the following is a weak opioid?

    A   ibuprofen
    B   codeine
    C   buprenorphine
    D   piroxicam
    E   morphine

4 Ms Qureshi has recently moved house and is experiencing dust allergy. She comes to the pharmacy to buy some *Clarityn* (loratadine). She is concerned about the side-effects of the drug. Which of the following is a side-effect?

    A   blurred vision
    B   fever
    C   bradycardia
    D   vomiting
    E   facial flushing

5 You are presented with the prescription opposite.
Taking all the drugs into consideration, from which disease is Mr Khan suffering?

    A   hypertension
    B   angina
    C   heart failure
    D   hyperlipidaemia
    E   arrhythmias

| Pharmacy stamp | Age<br><br>**34**<br><br>D.o.B.<br><br>**10/10/77** | Name (including forename) and address<br><br><br>S Khan<br><br>28 Ayraan St<br><br>London<br><br>WC1 |
|---|---|---|
| Number of days' treatment<br><br>N.B. Ensure dose is stated | | |

| Endorsements | | Office use |
|---|---|---|
| | Spironolactone 100 mg daily (28)<br>Enalapril 25 mg daily (28)<br>Bisoprolol 10 mg daily (28)<br>Digoxin 62.5 micrograms daily (28)<br>Furosemide 40 mg daily (28) | |

| Signature of doctor<br><br>*Nadia Bukhari* | In date |
|---|---|

| For<br><br>dispenser<br><br>No. of<br>persons<br>on form | **Dr N Bukhari**<br><br>**45 Handel House WC1**<br><br>**Brunswick Green PCT**<br><br>**97865430**<br><br>**Tel: 020 7753 5800** | FP10 C |
|---|---|---|

6    Which of the following colours the urine orange/red?

    A    ciprofloxacin
    B    amoxicillin
    C    rifampicin
    D    metronidazole
    E    oxytetracycline

7    You receive the following prescription in your pharmacy:

    Dianette sig 1 op
    Compression hosiery class I sig 1 pair
    Naproxen 500 mg sig 60

Assuming the patient pays for prescriptions, how many NHS charges are levied?

    A    1
    B    2
    C    3
    D    4
    E    5

8    Mrs Laher has been initiated on digoxin for heart failure. You monitor her urea and electrolytes daily. You notice one of her electrolyte levels is lower than it should be. This raises concern as low levels of the electrolyte may predispose to digoxin toxicity. Which electrolyte is of concern?

    A    sodium
    B    chloride
    C    magnesium
    D    potassium
    E    calcium

9    Mr Ahmed comes to your pharmacy with his first prescription for esmolol (beta-blocker). He asked to see you so that you could explain the side-effects of the drug. Which of the following is *not* a side-effect of esmolol?

    A    bradycardia
    B    fatigue
    C    coldness of the extremities
    D    urinary retention
    E    sexual dysfunction

10 The local GP wishes to prescribe a beta-blocker for hypertension for one of her patients, Nathan Warman. Nathan suffers from various other medical conditions. The GP asks for your advice as she is unsure whether a beta-blocker would be contraindicated in this patient. For which one of the following conditions are beta-blockers contraindicated?

    A    diabetes
    B    obesity
    C    pregnancy
    D    portal hypertension
    E    asthma

11 Z Rai is prescribed some amitriptyline tablets; which are classed as tricyclic antidepressants. You dispense the tablets and counsel her on the possible side-effects of the drug. Which of the following is *not* a side-effect of amitriptyline?

    A    constipation
    B    dry mouth
    C    drowsiness
    D    nystagmus
    E    urinary retention

12 Mr Ramsay is on a weight loss programme. He asks you, his pharmacist, to calculate his body mass index. Which of the following body mass index values indicates obesity?

    A    15
    B    23
    C    25
    D    29
    E    35

13 Mr Bukhari brings the prescription on the next page to your pharmacy: You advise him to take his medication during which part of the day?

    A    in the morning
    B    at lunchtime
    C    in the afternoon
    D    at teatime
    E    at bedtime

| Pharmacy stamp | Age<br><br>**31** | Name (including forename) and address<br><br>Taz Bukhari<br><br>86 Stanley Grove |
|---|---|---|
| Number of days' treatment<br><br>N.B. Ensure dose is stated | | London<br><br>N1 |
| Endorsements | Furosemide 40 mg<br><br>Sig. one od<br><br>Mitte 56 | Office use |
| Signature of doctor<br><br>*Nadia Bukhari* | In date | |
| NHS | PATIENTS – please read the notes overleaf | |

14   Mrs Khan has been prescribed GTN tablets for her angina attacks. She asks your advice on the side-effects that it may cause. Which of the following is *not* a side-effect of this drug?

A   facial flushing
B   throbbing headache
C   sleep disturbance
D   tachycardia
E   rash

15   Procyclidine is an antimuscarinic. Which of the following is *not* a side-effect of this drug?

A   urinary retention
B   dry mouth
C   diarrhoea
D   blurred vision
E   tachycardia

16   Mr Tim Renin is taking digoxin 250 micrograms daily as he has recently been diagnosed with atrial fibrillation. Which of the following is *not* a sign or symptom of digoxin toxicity?

A   dry mouth
B   bradycardia
C   vomiting
D   blurred vision
E   dizziness

17   Mr Munday is prescribed warfarin tablets at a recent outpatients' clinic. Which of the following is the correct indication for this drug?

A   analgesia
B   schizophrenia
C   hypertension
D   atrial fibrillation
E   Parkinson's disease

18   Ms Malik has been prescribed doxycyline 100 mg capsules for acne. Which of the following cautionary and advisory labels should be included on the final dispensed label?

A   with plenty of water
B   with food
C   dissolved under the tongue
D   sucked or chewed
E   half an hour before food

19   Ms Jamal has been diagnosed with schizophrenia for 2 years. The GP decides to introduce an intramuscular injection depot regimen to her treatment. How often should Ms Jamal receive her depot injection?

    A   once a year
    B   every 6 months
    C   every 1–4 weeks
    D   on alternate days
    E   once a day

20   Ms Mallick suffers with migraine. She comes to your pharmacy with the following drugs on her prescription:

    A   pizotifen
    B   fluoxetine
    C   *Microgynon*
    D   metoclopramide
    E   paracetamol

Which of the above drugs should be used with caution in this patient?

21   Which of the following antibiotics, if taken orally, should be taken an hour before food or on an empty stomach?

    A   flucloxacillin
    B   amoxicillin
    C   co-amoxiclav
    D   minocycline
    E   clindamycin

22   Mrs Pitt comes to see you at the pharmacy. She wants to start taking folic acid tablets as she's planning a pregnancy and has been told by her GP that it prevents neural tube defects in the fetus. What daily dose do you recommend for her?

    A   500 micrograms
    B   400 micrograms
    C   300 micrograms
    D   200 micrograms
    E   100 micrograms

**23** The following prescription is brought to your pharmacy.

| Pharmacy stamp | Age 42 | Name (including forename) and address Arif Lohar |
|---|---|---|
| Number of days' treatment N.B. Ensure dose is stated | 56 | 92 Langley Road London E17 |
| Endorsements | Rifampicin 450 mg daily Isoniazid 300 mg daily Ethambutol 300 mg Pyrazinamide 2 g daily | Office use |
| Signature of doctor *Nadia Bukhari* | In date | |
| NHS | PATIENTS – please read the notes overleaf | |

Looking at all the drugs the patient is prescribed, which of the following conditions does the patient suffer with?

    A    septicaemia
    B    cellulitis
    C    candidiasis
    D    tuberculosis
    E    HIV

24   Mr Hussain comes to your pharmacy as he has been severely sunburnt. You check his PMR and notice that one of his drugs causes phototoxicity. Which of the following requires him to use a wide-spectrum suncream?

   A   atenolol
   B   amiodarone
   C   enalapril
   D   ibuprofen
   E   senna

25   Ria Senn is prescribed ciprofloxacin for a chest infection. Which of the following drugs would have a potential interaction with this?

   A   ibuprofen
   B   propranolol
   C   simvastatin
   D   amoxicillin
   E   metformin

26   The following is written on a prescription:

   Nifedipine m/r 10 mg tablets
   Mitte 56
   Sig. one bd

You should advise the patient to:

   A   take the tablets after food
   B   avoid sunlight
   C   not stop taking the tablets unless advised by the doctor
   D   swallow the tablets whole and not chew them
   E   take the tablets sitting straight up

27   Which of the following may interact with simvastatin?

   A   cheese
   B   spinach
   C   salads
   D   olive oil
   E   grapefruit juice

28   Mrs Francis comes to your pharmacy to speak with you. She has read
     on the internet that omega-3 may improve her son's concentration. She
     had also read that omega-3 can be found in some types of fish. Which of
     the following fish contains the most omega-3?

    A   haddock
    B   salmon
    C   catfish
    D   cod
    E   shrimp

29   In the pharmacy, some drugs need to be stored in the fridge. What is the
     temperature range (in degrees celsius) for products to be stored in a
     fridge?

    A   −3–0
    B   0–3
    C   2–8
    D   3–9
    E   10–12

30   You are dispensing a cream in your pharmacy. The label states that the
     cream should be 'stored in a cool place'. Which of the following would
     be the correct storage temperature (in degrees celsius) for this?

    A   1
    B   3
    C   5
    D   9
    E   16

31   The prescription overleaf is not valid because:

    A   the patient's date of birth is missing
    B   the prescription is expired
    C   the number of days' treatment is missing
    D   the strength of the drug is missing
    E   the direction for taking the medication is missing

| Pharmacy stamp | Age | Name (including forename) and address |
|---|---|---|
| | **49** | Terry Tinkle |
| Number of days' treatment<br><br>N.B. Ensure dose is stated | | 125 Surbiton Lane<br><br>London<br><br>KT5 |
| *Endorsements* | Atorvastatin<br><br>Sig. One ON<br><br>56 tablets | *Office use* |
| Signature of doctor<br><br><br><br><br>*Nadia Bukhari* | In date<br><br>Balmoral Surgery<br><br>Balmoral Road<br><br>Surbiton KT5 | |
| NHS | PATIENTS – please read the notes overleaf | |

32    The prescription below is not legally valid because:

    A    the prescription is out of date
    B    the number of days' treatment is not included
    C    the patient's date of birth is missing
    D    the dose is missing
    E    the address of the doctor is missing

| Pharmacy stamp | Age | Name (including forename) and address |
|---|---|---|
| | **67** | Betsy Myers |
| Number of days' treatment<br><br>N.B. Ensure dose is stated | **28** | 1 Stanmore House<br><br>Southall<br><br>UB5 |
| Endorsements | Enalapril 10 mg<br><br>One daily | Office use |
| Signature of doctor<br><br>*Nadia Bukhari* | In date | |
| NHS | PATIENTS – please read the notes overleaf | |

33    How many prescription charges should Ms Boop be charged?

    A    0
    B    1
    C    2
    D    3
    E    4

| Pharmacy stamp | Age 29 | Name (including forename) and address B Boop 57 Redbridge Road London E17 |
|---|---|---|
| Number of days' treatment N.B. Ensure dose is stated | | |
| Endorsements | Micronor 3 x 28 Take one daily | Office use |
| Signature of Doctor *Nadia Bukhari* | In date Balmoral Surgery Balmoral Road Surbiton KT5 | |
| NHS | PATIENTS – please read the notes overleaf | |

**34** How many times should Mr Abraham's prescription be dispensed?

        **A**   1
        **B**   2
        **C**   3
        **D**   4
        **E**   5

| *Pharmacy Stamp* | Age | Name (including forename) and address |
|---|---|---|
| | **21** | John Abraham |
| Number of days' treatment<br><br>N.B. Ensure dose is stated | | 123 Tooting Hill Grove<br><br>Tooting<br><br>SW17 |
| *Endorsements* | Fluoxetine 20 mg<br><br>Take one in the morning<br><br>Mitte 30<br><br>Repeat 3 times | *Office use* |
| Signature of doctor<br><br>*Nadia Bukhari* | In date<br><br>Balmoral Surgery<br><br>Balmoral Road<br><br>Surbiton KT5 | |
| NHS | PATIENTS – please read the notes overleaf | |

35 How many lansoprazole capsules will you dispense for Mr Smith?

     A   2
     B   14
     C   28
     D   56
     E   72

| Pharmacy Stamp | Age | Name (including forename) and address |
|---|---|---|
| | **35** | George Smith |
| Number of days' treatment<br><br>N.B. Ensure dose is stated | 28 | 25 Acre Road<br><br>Kingston KT2 |
| Endorsements | Lansoprazole 15 mg<br><br>Sig om, and on | Office use |
| Signature of doctor<br><br>*Nadia Bukhari* | In date<br><br>Balmoral Surgery<br><br>Balmoral Road<br><br>Surbiton KT5 | |
| NHS | PATIENTS – please read the notes overleaf | |

36   Mr Williams comes to your pharmacy for an emergency supply of captopril tablets, which he regularly takes. You dispense the emergency supply to him and label the product. Which of the following is not a requirement for the emergency supply dispensed label?

    A   the date of dispensing
    B   the address of the doctor
    C   the words 'emergency supply'
    D   the total quantity of tablets dispensed
    E   the address of the pharmacy at which it was dispensed

37   Ms Pin Luk comes to your pharmacy for an emergency supply of her *Microgynon* oral contraceptive pill. She takes it every morning before she goes to work and has run out without realising. You decide to dispense the emergency supply. How many tablets do you dispense?

    A   1
    B   5
    C   7
    D   10
    E   21

38   Which of the following is incorrect with respect to schedule 2 controlled drugs?

    A   A record must be made in the controlled drug register
    B   A doctor may administer the drug
    C   The prescription is valid for 13 weeks
    D   The address of the prescriber must be in the UK
    E   Invoices do not need to be retained for 2 years

39   Which of the following is incorrect with respect to temazepam?

    A   It is a schedule 4 controlled drug
    B   Invoices need to be retained for 2 years
    C   It needs to be stored under the Safe Custody regulations
    D   A licence is required if you wish to export it
    E   It does not subject to controlled drug prescription requirements

40 With respect to record-keeping requirements of schedule 2 controlled drugs, which is false?

    A   Records must be kept in a register

    B   The pharmacist does not need to record whether the person collecting is the patient, a representative or a healthcare professional

    C   If a healthcare professional is collecting, his or her name and address must be recorded

    D   Proof of identity provided by the person collecting must be recorded

    E   The pharmacist must confirm the identity of the person collecting the CD

41 Which of the following drugs is classed as a beta-blocker?

    A   captopril

    B   sotalol

    C   simvastatin

    D   furosemide

    E   digoxin

42 Which of the following may *not* cause a dry cough as an adverse drug reaction?

    A   enalapril

    B   lisinopril

    C   ramipril

    D   losartan

    E   captopril

43 Which of the following may cause hypokalaemia?

    A   spironalactone

    B   furosemide

    C   bendroflumethiazide

    D   bumetanide

    E   chlortalidone

**44** Which of the following foods has a high vitamin K content?

    **A** bananas
    **B** fish
    **C** spinach
    **D** apples
    **E** milk

**45** Which of the following is classed as an antiplatelet drug?

    **A** lansoprazole
    **B** cimetidine
    **C** clopidogrel
    **D** paracetamol
    **E** warfarin

**46** Which of the following is a narrow therapeutic index drug and requires therapeutic dose monitoring?

    **A** ciclosporin
    **B** propranolol
    **C** beclomethasone
    **D** pravastatin
    **E** perindopril

**47** Which of the following may cause a fine tremor as an adverse effect?

    **A** beclomethasone
    **B** salbutamol
    **C** theophylline
    **D** senna
    **E** ipratropium bromide

**48** Which of the following should you counsel the patient to take with or after food?

    **A** paracetamol
    **B** atenolol
    **C** naproxen
    **D** fluoxetine
    **E** amoxicillin

49  Which of the following is prescribed first-line in type 2 diabetes for obese patients?

   A   glibenclamide
   B   metformin
   C   glipizide
   D   rosiglitazone
   E   acarbose

50  Gentamicin is an aminoglycoside. Which of the following is a toxic effect of this drug?

   A   hepatotoxicity
   B   ototoxicity
   C   hyperkalaemia
   D   closed-angle glaucoma
   E   endocarditis

51  A preterm baby is defined as having completed:

   A   less than 37 weeks of gestation
   B   less than 38 weeks of gestation
   C   less than 39 weeks of gestation
   D   less than 40 weeks of gestation
   E   less than 42 weeks of gestation

52  Pyrexia in children under the age of 5 years is defined as:

   A   body temperature of 32°C
   B   body temperature of 36°C
   C   body temperature of 36.6°C
   D   body temperature of 37°C
   E   body temperature of 37.6°C

53  You receive a prescription for the following item:

   Drug X Troch.
   Use as directed
   Mitte ×1 OP
What does 'Troch.' stand for?

   A   tablet
   B   oro-dispersible tablet
   C   inhaler
   D   triple pack
   E   lozenge

54   Which one of the following predisposes patients to oral thrush?

    A   *Bambec* tablets
    B   *En-De-Kay* tablets
    C   *Oxis Turbohaler*
    D   *Corlan* pellets
    E   *Daktarin* oral gel

55   Asian ginseng is traditionally used for:

    A   menorrhagia
    B   irritable bowel syndrome
    C   weight loss
    D   sleeping aid
    E   improvement of the immune system

56   A 26-year-old woman is going on holiday and is worried she may develop diarrhoea. She asks you to recommend something. Which of the following is the first-line treatment for acute diarrhoea?

    A   vancomycin
    B   kaolin and morphine
    C   loperamide
    D   oral rehydration salts
    E   hyoscine butylbromide

57   Which of the following describes a localised collection of blood, usually clotted, in an organ, space or tissue?

    A   haematoma
    B   haematemesis
    C   haematuria
    D   haematocrit
    E   haemophilia

58   Which of the following is defined as an open comedone?

    A   papule
    B   blackhead
    C   whitehead
    D   acne cyst
    E   pustule

59    Which of the following products sold in the pharmacy is the least likely to be abused?

    **A**   *Sinutab*
    **B**   *Pardale-V* tablets
    **C**   Glycerol suppositories
    **D**   *Robitussin* chesty cough syrup
    **E**   *Vicks Medinite*

60    Which of the following *cannot* request an emergency supply of a prescription-only medicine?

    **A**   Swiss doctor
    **B**   dentist
    **C**   vet
    **D**   supplementary nurse prescriber
    **E**   community nurse prescriber

61    Mr W is a regular patient of yours and comes into your pharmacy to collect his weekly instalment of methadone. He returns, 30 minutes later, asking for another to be dispensed as he tripped and broke the bottle containing methadone. He shows you the bump on his head. Which of the following is the most appropriate response?

    **A**   Dispense next week's methadone but contact his prescriber to obtain a prescription for next week's instalment
    **B**   Tell him there's nothing you can do about it and refer him to the nearest accident and emergency department
    **C**   Find out more details about the area where he dropped the bottle and send a member of staff to confirm his story. If it is true, supply another bottle
    **D**   Advise Mr W that he must go back to his prescriber to request another prescription
    **E**   Inform Mr W that you must contact the police and prescriber before dispensing any more methadone to him

62    Under the NHS contract, which of the following is an advanced service?

    **A**   repeat dispensing
    **B**   needle and syringe exchange
    **C**   medicines use review and prescription intervention service
    **D**   minor ailment service
    **E**   patient group directions

63 Regarding the Hazardous Waste Regulations 2005 in England and Wales, which of the following should a registered pharmacy *not* accept (assuming it does not have a licence from the Environmental Agency)?

    A    medicinal waste from a residential care home
    B    methadone from a patient's representative
    C    expired methotrexate
    D    industrial waste
    E    waste from a caravan

64 Which one of the following expired dispensary stock does *not* need to be destroyed in the presence of an authorised witness?

    A    benzfetamine
    B    pethidine
    C    methylphenidate
    D    morphine
    E    oripavine

65 All of the following patients have recently had unprotected sex. Assuming there are no other contraindications, to which one of the following patients can you supply emergency hormonal contraception without referral?

    A    a 29-year-old woman whose period is abnormally light
    B    an 18-year-old woman who suffers from unstable angina
    C    a 17-year-old girl who had unprotected sex 42 hours ago
    D    a 28-year-old woman who bleeds between her periods
    E    a 36-year-old whose period is 4 days late

66 Which of the following should a pharmacist *not* do when conducting a pregnancy test?

    A    Obtain a request for the test which is signed and dated by the patient
    B    Record the answers for all of the questions asked, test results and types of test used and their batch number
    C    Provide the results in writing on a standardised form
    D    At the patient's request, send a copy of the form to her doctor
    E    Carry out the test in the dispensary sink

67   Faulty medical devices should be reported to:

  A   General Pharmaceutical Council
  B   Medicines and Healthcare products Regulatory Agency
  C   National Institute for Health and Clinical Excellence
  D   National Patient Safety Agency
  E   Pharmaceutical Services Negotiating Committee

68   Regarding counterfeit medicines, which of the following is *incorrect*?

  A   Report suspected counterfeit medicines to the MHRA immediately
  B   Inform the patients and other pharmacy branches of the suspected counterfeit medicines
  C   In response to a drug alert, return any counterfeit medicines as outlined in the guidance and search the PMR for patients who may have received the counterfeit medicines to take the necessary action
  D   If a patient suspects that he/she may have a counterfeit drug you should record the patient's contact details, reason for patient's suspicion, product name, dosage, batch number and expiry date and inform the relevant agency immediately
  E   Altered expiry dates, cheap bulk sales and breaks or tears in the packaging are all good indicators for counterfeit medicines

69   Legislation permits pharmacists who are providing services to drug misusers to supply specific drug paraphernalia to illicit drug users. Which of the following items is *not* permitted to be supplied?

  A   3 mL ampoules of sterile water for injection
  B   swabs
  C   a spoon
  D   ascorbic acid
  E   filters

70   What does the 'CE' mark stand for on licensed devices?

  A   checked for excellence
  B   created in England
  C   compounded in Europe
  D   company establishment
  E   *conformité européenne*

**71** Patients taking the following drugs should immediately report to their doctors if they develop a sore throat. Which one of the following drugs does this warning *not* apply to?

    **A** carbimazole
    **B** carbamazepine
    **C** phenytoin
    **D** misoprostol
    **E** methotrexate

**72** Which of the following classes of drugs is *unlikely* to cause nausea and/or vomiting as a side-effect?

    **A** vinca alkaloids
    **B** phenothiazines
    **C** cardiac glycosides
    **D** sulphonylureas
    **E** macrolide antibiotics

**73** Which of the following drugs is *not* hepatotoxic?

    **A** azathioprine
    **B** digoxin
    **C** isoniazid
    **D** rifampicin
    **E** sodium valproate

**74** A client purchases a *Paludrine/Avloclor* travel pack after being interviewed by the pharmacist. How long before and after travelling to the endemic area should prophylaxis against malaria be taken?

    **A** 1–2 days before travel, during the stay and for 4 weeks after return
    **B** 1–2 days before travel, during the stay and for 1 week after return
    **C** 1 week before travel, during the stay and for 4 weeks after return
    **D** 1 week before travel, during the stay and for 6 weeks after return
    **E** 2–3 weeks before travel, during the stay and for 1 week after return

75 Which one of the following is least likely to trigger a migraine attack?

    A   *Femodene*
    B   menopause
    C   depression
    D   bupropion
    E   obesity

76 Which of the following side-effects is *not* associated with the corresponding drug?

    A   unexplained bruising with methotrexate
    B   gynaecomastia with amitriptyline
    C   oral thrush with betamethasone inhaler
    D   hypokalaemia with prednisolone
    E   constipation with ciprofloxacin

77 A worried mother requests your advice about itchy, seeping spots that have developed around her daughter's mouth. After questioning you find out that her daughter is 5 years old and that the spots were preceded by a small red itchy patch of inflamed skin. What is the most appropriate course of action to take?

    A   Her child may have chickenpox: supply calamine lotion and advise her to keep her child off school and to maintain hygiene measures, e.g. to cut the child's nails
    B   Her child may have impetigo: refer her to the doctor. Advise her to keep her child off school as she is currently contagious and to maintain hygiene, e.g. do not share towels
    C   Her child may have rubella: refer her immediately to the doctor
    D   Her child may have measles: refer her immediately to the doctor
    E   Her child may have developed an allergy to food

78 Which one of the following drug does *not* colour bodily secretions?

    A   triamterene
    B   clioquinol
    C   levodopa
    D   co-danthramer
    E   rifampicin

79    Which one of the following does *not* need to be stored at 2–8°C?

    A    *Proctosedyl* suppositories
    B    *Daktacort* cream (30 g)
    C    *Revaxis* (diphtheria, tetanus and polio) vaccine
    D    *Humulin M3* pen (in-use)
    E    *Duac Once Daily*

80    For which of the following drugs do patients *not* need to carry an alert card?

    A    steroids
    B    lithium
    C    oxygen
    D    warfarin
    E    phenytoin

81    You should avoid direct contact with all of the following except:

    A    methotrexate
    B    finasteride
    C    doxycycline
    D    oestradiol
    E    chlorpromazine hydrochloride

82    To which one of the following patients would it be appropriate to sell 400 microgram tamsulosin hydrochloride tablets (assuming there are no other contraindications)?

    A    a 23-year-old man who frequently gets up during the night to urinate and is excessively thirsty
    B    a 48-year-old man who has difficulty urinating, is constantly tired and has shortness of breath
    C    a 72-year-old man who finds it difficult to start and urinates very frequently
    D    a 56-year-old man who is currently taking indoramin for his high blood pressure
    E    a woman who is experiencing pain on urination

83    The symbol $\boxed{\text{NHS}}$ next to a drug's name means:

    A   not available in hospitals
    B   community nurse prescribers cannot prescribe
    C   doctors cannot prescribe
    D   less suitable for prescribing on the NHS
    E   this preparation cannot be prescribed on the NHS

84    For the treatment of overdose, which one of the following combinations is incorrect?

    A   warfarin and phytomenadione
    B   heparin and protamine
    C   paracetamol and acetylcysteine
    D   morphine and naloxone
    E   lithium and sodium bicarbonate

85    Which one of the following is a common sign of digoxin toxicity?

    A   nystagmus
    B   tachycardia
    C   visual disturbances
    D   jaundice
    E   convulsions

86    Assuming there are no other contraindications, you can sell *Alli* to a person with which body mass index?

    A   $18\,kg/m^2$
    B   $22\,kg/m^2$
    C   $25\,kg/m^2$
    D   $27\,kg/m^2$
    E   $30\,kg/m^2$

87    Which of the following drugs should be avoided in patients with active liver disease?

    A   lithium
    B   prazosin
    C   digoxin
    D   ketoconazole
    E   metoclopramide

88  A 16-year-old boy asks for your advice about an itchy rash which he has developed on his arm. After questioning him further you find out that he has recently started working in a pet shop and that the rash started as a small red spot which spread outwards. It now looks like an inflamed ring of skin with a healed centre. Which of the following skin conditions is this most likely to be?

  A   contact dermatitis
  B   herpes simplex
  C   impetigo
  D   ringworm
  E   roundworm

89  Which of the following drugs is *not* a suitable treatment for an acute gout attack?

  A   colchicine
  B   indometacin
  C   ketoprofen
  D   allopurinol
  E   naproxen

90  Which one of the following is *not* a sign or symptom of cocaine abuse?

  A   agitation
  B   dilated pupils
  C   muscle tension
  D   hypertension
  E   bradycardia

91  Which of the following drugs is *not* known to increase the risk of bleeding when taken concomitantly with aspirin?

  A   citalopram
  B   mefenamic acid
  C   indoramin
  D   venlafaxine
  E   warfarin

92 For which of the following drugs does the brand name *not* need to be specified on the prescription?

    A   theophylline m/r capsules
    B   phenytoin tablets
    C   lithium tablets
    D   diltiazem m/r tablets
    E   digoxin tablets

93 Some drugs have side-effects which affect the patient's ability to drive or operate machinery safely. Which of the following drugs does *not* have this effect?

    A   zopiclone
    B   chlorpromazine
    C   loratadine
    D   tamsulosin hydrochloride
    E   prednisolone

94 Which of the following is the recommended limit for drinking alcohol?

    A   Men should not exceed 21 units per day and women should not exceed 14 units per day on a regular basis
    B   Men should not exceed 3–4 units per day and women should not exceed 2–3 units per day on a regular basis
    C   Men should not exceed 6 units per day and women should not exceed 4 units per day on a regular basis
    D   Men should not exceed 10 units per day and women should not exceed 5 units per day on a regular basis
    E   Both men and women should not exceed 4 units per day on a regular basis

95 Dull pain or discomfort in the right upper quadrant may indicate the presence of:

    A   diverticulitis
    B   IBS
    C   appendicitis
    D   hepatitis
    E   pyelonephritis

96 Which of the following drugs is known to affect the absorption of vitamin D?

    A   metformin
    B   isoniazid
    C   rosuvastatin
    D   colestyramine
    E   lithium

97 Which one of the following preparations can cause rhinitis medicamentosa with prolonged use?

    A   saline nasal drops
    B   pseudoephedrine tablets
    C   chlorphenamine syrup
    D   fluticasone nasal spray
    E   oxymetazoline nasal spray

98 Which one of the following patients is *not* exempt from paying NHS prescription charges?

    A   a 17-year-old girl with a prescription for naproxen 500 mg tablets in Scotland
    B   a 53-year-old woman with a prescription for anastrozole tablets in England
    C   a 58-year-old man with a prescription for goserelin implant in England
    D   a 30-year-old woman with a prescription for *TT380* Slimline IUD in England
    E   a 20-year-old man with a prescription for *Proscar* tablets in Wales

99 Which of the following pharmacy products is *not* licensed as a medical device?

    A   test strips
    B   condoms
    C   dressings
    D   thermometers
    E   creams and ointments

100 Pharmacy contractors who have not received discount to specific listed items will not have discount deducted in respect of NHS prescription reimbursement. Which of the following drug classes are *not* classed as 'discount not given' (DNG)?

    A   cold-chain items
    B   cytotoxic or cytostatic items
    C   insulins for injection
    D   vaccines
    E   appliances

101 All of the following drugs can be prescribed on NHS prescriptions for the stated purpose and must include the reference SLS, except which one of the following?

    A   clobazam for epilepsy
    B   cyanocobalamin tablets for the prevention of vitamin $B_{12}$ deficiency
    C   *Cialis* for the treatment of erectile dysfunction
    D   *Relenza* for the treatment of influenza
    E   minoxidil topical solution for alopecia

102 Mr B is *not* exempt from paying NHS prescription charges. He presents you with a prescription for *Tegretol* 100 mg and *Tegretol Retard* 400 mg tablets. How many charges will you take from him?

    A   no charge
    B   1 charge
    C   2 charges
    D   3 charges
    E   4 charges

103 Which one of the following combined oral contraceptives may be used to treat severe acne in women?

    A   norgestimate with ethinylestradiol
    B   gestodene with ethinylestradiol
    C   cyproterone acetate with ethinylestradiol
    D   drospirenone with ethinylestradiol
    E   desogestrel with ethinylestradiol

*The answers for this section are on pp. 137–148.*

## MULTIPLE COMPLETION QUESTIONS

Each one of the questions or incomplete statements in this section is followed by three responses. For each question, ONE or MORE of the responses is/are correct. Decide which of the responses is/are correct, then choose:

A　　if **1, 2** and **3** are correct
B　　if **1** and **2** only are correct
C　　if **2** and **3** only are correct
D　　if **1** only is correct
E　　if **3** only is correct

| Summary | | | | |
|---|---|---|---|---|
| A | B | C | D | E |
| 1, 2, 3 | 1, 2 only | 2, 3 only | 1 only | 3 only |

1　　Which of the following is/are considered to be a pharmacodynamic interaction?

　　1　captopril + atenolol
　　2　propranol + amlodipine
　　3　ibuprofen + furosemide

2　　Which of the following is/are considered to be a pharmacokinetic interaction?

　　1　lithium + ibuprofen
　　2　warfarin + aspirin
　　3　salbutamol + bendroflumethiazide

3　　Which of the following is/are not a side-effect of insulin?

　　1　hypoglycaemia
　　2　taste disturbance
　　3　black stools

4    Miss Rai takes *Yasmin*, a combined oral contraceptive pill, regularly and would like to know possible side-effects. Which of the following is/are side-effects?

1    migraine
2    abdominal cramps
3    liver impairment

5    Mr North has recently been diagnosed with hypothyroidism. Which of the following is/are appropriate to prescribe for this condition?

1    carbimazole
2    prednisolone
3    levothyroxine

6    Mrs Demetri has been recommended to buy malathion liquid over the counter by her pharmacist. Choose from the following the condition(s) for which this may be counter-prescribed.

1    crab lice
2    head lice
3    threadworm

7    Mrs Naqvi has been prescribed prednisolone for long-term treatment. Which of the following is/are side-effects that Mrs Naqvi may experience?

1    osteoporosis
2    glaucoma
3    diabetes

8    Which of the following is/are used predominantly for their glucocorticoid activity?

1    betamethasone
2    hydrocortisone
3    fludrocortisone

9    Mr Tomlin suffers with type 2 diabetes. He regularly visits a diabetic clinic. Which of the following parameters should be monitored regularly in type 2 diabetic patients?

1    glycosylated haemoglobin
2    blood glucose concentration
3    urine protein concentration

10   Which of the following parameters *only* demonstrate(s) *long-term* glycaemic control in diabetic patients?

1   blood glucose concentration
2   urine ketone concentration
3   glycosylated haemoglobin

11   Mr Haydon is going travelling for a year. One of his destinations is Pakistan. He comes to your pharmacy for some antimalaria advice. Which of the following is/are suitable for the prophylaxis of malaria?

1   proguanil hydrochloride
2   chloroquine
3   doxycycline

12   Miss Kantaria comes to the pharmacy complaining of vaginal candidiasis. Assuming she is not taking any other medication or suffering with any illness, which of the following can be counter-prescribed for this patient?

1   *Diflucan One* capsule
2   *Canesten* pessaries
3   nystatin suspension

13   Ms Issac is suffering with a urinary tract infection. Which of the following antibiotics is/are appropriate to prescribe for such a condition?

1   metronidazole
2   trimethroprim
3   nitrofurantoin

14   Mr Pearce is a patient on your ward suffering with endocarditis. The microbiology team recommend that he is prescribed vancomycin for this. You are aware that this drug requires therapeutic dose monitoring. Which of the following is/are toxic effects of this drug?

1   ototoxicity
2   nephrotoxicity
3   hepatotoxicity

15   Which of the following is/are true with respect to tetracycline?

1   It should *not* be prescribed for children under 12 years
2   It should *not* be given to pregnant women
3   It should *not* be given to patients with renal impairment

16 Which of the following drugs is/are indicated for neuropathic pain?

1 gabapentin
2 ibuprofen
3 morphine

17 Which statement(s) is/are true with regards to morphine?

1 It is classed as a strong opioid
2 It may cause respiratory depression
3 It is a schedule 1 controlled drug

18 Which of the following is/are classed as an oral antidiabetic drug?

1 acarbose
2 glucagon
3 diazoxide

19 Which of the following is/are true with respect to emergency supply at the request of a doctor?

1 The prescription must be sent to the pharmacist dispensing the emergency supply within 96 hours
2 The prescription-only medicine may be a schedule 2 controlled drug
3 An entry in the prescription-only register must be made on the day of the supply or the next day if impractical on the same day

20 With respect to pharmacist supplementary prescribers, a clinical management plan must state the following:

1 the name of the patient
2 circumstances in which the supplementary prescriber should refer to or seek advice from the doctor
3 the date the plan takes effect

21 Which of the following persons is/are permitted to supply or administer under a patient group direction?

1 registered nurses
2 dental hygienists
3 registered speech and language therapists

22  Which is/are true with respect to facsimile transmission of prescriptions?

    1    A fax is a legally valid prescription

    2    Any doubt about the content of the original prescription caused by poor reproduction must be clarified prior to dispensing

    3    Schedule 3 controlled drugs cannot be dispensed against a fax

23  Which is/are true with regard to dentists prescribing?

    1    They must be prescribed on a FP10D form for NHS patients

    2    A dental prescription is valid under the Medicines Act 1968, even though the item prescribed is *not* on the Dental Practitioners' Formulary

    3    A dentist cannot make an emergency supply request

24  Which of the following is/are pharmacy-only (P) medicines?

    1    paracetamol 500 mg 16 tablets

    2    ibuprofen 200 mg 16 tablets

    3    ranitidine 75 mg 7 tablets

25  Which of the following is/are a general sales list (GSL) item?

    1    almond oil

    2    *Beconase* hayfever nasal spray

    3    *Dentinox* teething gel

26  Which of the following is/are a prescription-only medicine (POM)?

    1    amoxicillin 500 mg capsules

    2    GTN 300 microgram tablets

    3    *Oilatum* gel

27  Which of the following is/are *not* a GSL item?

    1    paracetamol 500 mg tablets × 100

    2    *Ovex* tablets × 4

    3    paraffin white and yellow soft BP

28  Which of the following is/are *not* a P item?

    1    phenytoin tablets

    2    atenolol tablets

    3    piroxicam capsules

29 Which of the following is/are *not* a POM item?

    1    *Lemsip Max* capsules
    2    Infadrops
    3    *Meltus* baby cough linctus

30 Which of the following is/are significant drug interactions (black dot interactions) in the BNF?

    1    atenolol + furosemide
    2    digoxin + bendroflumethiazide
    3    diltiazem + bumetanide

31 A patient who presents with which of the following symptoms should be advised to seek immediate medical attention?

    1    melaena
    2    haemoptysis
    3    haematemesis

32 What causes halitosis?

    1    sinusitis
    2    gingivitis
    3    smoking

33 Impetigo is caused by which of the following bacteria?

    1    *Staphylococcus aureus*
    2    *Streptococcus pyogenes*
    3    *Streptococcus agalactiae*

34 Which of the following is/are basic requirements that a Society inspector will look for during his/her routine visit to a registered pharmacy?

    1    The fridge must contain a maximum/minimum thermometer
    2    The statutory notice 'Now clean your hands' must be displayed in the toilet area
    3    The dispensary sink should provide drinkable water which is clearly marked for that purpose

35   In the detection of a forged prescription, pharmacists should be aware of:

1   prescription-only medicines which are especially subject to misuse, e.g. steroids
2   'Dr' before or after the prescriber's signature
3   excessive quantities of any medicine

36   The Code of Ethics requires all registered pharmacy professionals to develop their knowledge and competence in their area of practice. Which of the following is/are true in relation to CPD?

1   It is a mandatory requirement to complete a minimum of 7 CPD entries every 12 months
2   All entries must be submitted on RPSGB-approved forms
3   Shadowing a colleague can be an example of CPD

37   You receive the following FP10MDA prescription:

Methadone hydrochloride 1 mg/mL syrup
30 mL once daily
Supply 420 mL (four hundred and twenty millilitres)
Supervised consumption, 30 mL every day from Monday to Saturday. Dispense Sunday's dose on Saturday

Which of the following is/are true?

1   Instalment prescriptions must have *both* the dose and instalment amount stated separately
2   Schedule 2, 3 and 4 part II must be denatured before disposal
3   Cocaine, diamorphine or diethylpropion can only be administered by a specially authorised doctor who holds a Home Office licence

38   Pharmacists should be aware of the following correct statement(s), regarding controlled drugs:

1   The first instalment or the first batch of a repeat prescription must be dispensed within 28 days of the appropriate prescription date
2   It is good practice to contact the prescriber of a schedule 2, 3 or 4 controlled drug if the supply exceeds 30 days
3   Repeat prescriptions for schedules 3 and 4 are allowed on the NHS

39  Which of the following actions/procedures contribute to the continuous improvement of quality and maintenance of high standards of NHS services?

1   audit on procedures to deal with poor performance
2   incidence report forms and error reviews
3   local patient feedback questionnaires

40  A practising pharmacist who receives a criminal conviction must inform which of the following?

1   the General Pharmaceutical Council
2   his or her employer
3   none of the above, as the convictions are a personal matter

41  Regarding clinical audits, which of the following statements is/are true?

1   Clinical audits are part of clinical governance
2   A community pharmacy is required to complete at least two clinical audits annually
3   A clinical audit is a continuous cycle of reflection, planning, action and evaluation

42  A private prescription for *Subutex*:

1   must be written on a standardised form which is sent to the relevant NHS agency and contain the prescriber's identification number
2   must state the dose, form, strength and quantity (in both words and figures)
3   can be dispensed as instalments or repeatable batches

43  The Royal Pharmaceutical Society's guidance on developing and implementing standard operating procedures (SOPs) for dispensing states:

1   The name of the pharmacist under whose authority the SOP was prepared should be clearly specified
2   The requirement to put in place and implement dispensing SOPs does not apply to pharmacies with no dispensary support staff
3   SOPs must be followed at all times regardless of a change in circumstances

44      Mrs F is a regular methadone client. She picks up her prescription once weekly and always brings her son with her. Her son is a very active child who usually rushes to your staff to tell them of his recent adventures. During his next visit you notice a bruise on his forehead and when you approach him to start a conversation he runs behind his mother's legs looking petrified. Which of the following actions is/are the most appropriate?

     1      Discuss your concerns with the named professional for child protection or the designated member of staff within your organisation, the PCT or the Health Board

     2      Keep records of your concerns and any actions which you take

     3      Confront Mrs F, as it is unlikely that she would have physically abused her child, and offer to help

45      The personal and professional conduct of a registered pharmacist is measured against the seven principles of the code of ethics. Which of the following is/are part of the seven principles?

     1      Show respect for others

     2      Develop your professional knowledge and competence

     3      Encourage patients to participate in decisions about their care

46      It is 6 p.m. on a bank holiday weekend and Mrs E, your local vet, telephones you to request an emergency supply of insulin for her patient's cat. She assures you that she will supply you with a veterinary prescription on Tuesday morning. Regarding emergency supplies, which of the following statements is/are true?

     1      Pharmacists should be satisfied that there is an immediate need for the medication

     2      Prescribers must issue a prescription within 72 hours of the request

     3      You may supply the insulin in response to Mrs E's request

47      The following statement(s) is/are true with regard to unlicensed medicines:

     1      They are medicines without a UK marketing authorisation and include specials, repackaged medicines and extemporaneous preparations

     2      They can be prescribed by a dentist

     3      Records relating to their supply must be kept for 5 years

48 Regarding metronidazole, which of the following statements is/are true?

   1    It is an antimicrobial drug with high activity against anaerobic bacteria and protozoa

   2    Alcohol consumption should be avoided during and for 48 hours after administration

   3    It can be used to treat *Clostridium difficile* infection caused by treatment with amoxicillin

49 Which of the following statements is/are true regarding the shelf-life of medicines?

   1    Reconstituted *Zineryt* has a shelf-life of 5 weeks

   2    After opening, *Persantin* has a shelf-life of 6 weeks

   3    After opening, glyceryl trinitrate long-acting tablets have a shelf-life of 8 weeks

50 Regarding lipophilic drugs, which of the following statements is/are true?

   1    They readily penetrate the blood–brain barrier

   2    They have a high apparent volume of distribution

   3    They are readily excreted unchanged from the kidneys

51 You dispense a new prescription for Mr G, a regular patient. The prescription reads:

> Allopurinol 100 mg tablets
> Take one daily
> Mitte 28 tablets

Which of the following counselling points would you give to Mr G?

   1    Take after food

   2    Take with plenty of water

   3    Do not stop taking this medicine except on your doctor's advice

52 Mrs J is a 24-year-old woman who has recently been diagnosed with schizophrenia. She is prescribed an antipsychotic depot injection. Regarding this type of injection, which of the following statements is/are true?

   1    Long-acting preparations are preferred in patients who are non-compliant with oral antipsychotics

   2    They are administered by deep intramuscular injection at intervals of 1–4 weeks

   3    Oral typical antipsychotics are more likely to cause extrapyramidal symptoms than depot injections

53  For which of the following drugs must you ensure that the dispensed brand is the same as the patient has previously been taking?

1  nifedipine m/r
2  diltiazem LA
3  carbamazepine

54  Regarding beta-blockers, the following statement(s) is/are correct:

1  They can be used in thyrotoxicosis, angina, migraine and anxiety
2  Side-effects include fatigue, coldness of the extremities and sleep disturbances with nightmares
3  They have the advisory label 'do not stop taking this medicine except on your doctor's advice'

55  Regarding lithium, the following statement(s) is/are *incorrect*:

1  The concomitant administration of diuretics, NSAIDs or ACE inhibitors reduces the excretion of lithium and thus increases the risk of toxicity
2  Patients should maintain an adequate fluid intake and should avoid dietary changes which might reduce or increase sodium intake
3  Prescribing lithium generically is good practice

56  Which of the following patients is/are at higher risk of developing peripheral neuropathy with isoniazid?

1  a person with HIV infection
2  an individual suffering from anorexia
3  an alcoholic

57  When presented with the following ailments in community pharmacy, which should you refer to a medical practitioner and *not* treat with OTC medications?

1  a 46-year-old man who finds it difficult to urinate
2  a 17-year-old boy who has thrush, is excessively thirsty and has unexpectedly lost weight
3  a 57-year-old man with dyspepsia which has *not* responded to OTC products

58  On Monday morning, Mr W presents you with a prescription for *Deximune* (ciclosporin) 25 mg capsules. You search your stock and find that you only have *Neoral* 25 mg capsules in stock. Which of the following actions do you take?

    1  Ask the prescriber to change the prescription to '*Neoral* 25 mg capsules'

    2  Dispense and endorse the prescription with *Neoral* 25 mg capsules

    3  Order *Deximune* 25 mg capsules for this patient

59  Regarding treatment with amiodarone, which of the following statements is/are true?

    1  Common side-effects include taste disturbances, tremor and sleep disorders

    2  Patients should be told to notify their medical practitioner immediately if they develop a persistent dry cough and shortness of breath

    3  Stop treatment if hypothyroidism or severe hepatic impairment develops

60  The serum concentrations of theophylline may reach subtherapeutic levels when administered concomitantly with which of the following drugs?

    1  St John's wort

    2  verapamil

    3  erythromycin

61  Which of the following drugs is/are likely to cause diarrhoea?

    1  digoxin

    2  magnesium trisilicate

    3  pethidine hydrochloride

62  Mrs P regularly picks up her medication (*Marvelon*) from your pharmacy. The next time you see her, she presents you with a prescription that has additional drugs. For which of the following drugs should you advise her to take extra contraceptive precautions?

    1  griseofulvin

    2  olanzapine

    3  digoxin

63 Which of the following antibiotics can be used to treat a lower urinary tract infection?

1 ciprofloxacin
2 trimethoprim
3 nitrofurantoin

64 Regarding oral penicillins, which of the following statements is/are true?

1 A person who is allergic to one penicillin will be allergic to all other penicillins
2 Anaphylactic reactions occur in 1–10% of treated individuals
3 A rash that occurs more than 24 hours after penicillin administration is not considered to be a penicillin allergy

65 Mr H is a 27-year-old man who is taking phenelzine. Which of the following foods should he avoid?

1 yeast extract (e.g. *Marmite*)
2 mature cheese
3 low-alcohol drinks

66 Regarding liver failure, which of the following statements is/are true?

1 Drugs which may damage the liver include rosuvastatin and methotrexate
2 People who are at risk of liver toxicity should immediately report the following symptoms to their doctor: nausea, vomiting, abdominal discomfort and dark urine
3 Lactulose can be used to decrease bacterial growth in hepatic encephalopathy

67 You should not sell aspirin to patients who:

1 are taking methotrexate
2 are G6PD-deficient
3 developed hives after using *Voltarol*

68 Which of the following drugs is/are allowed to be issued by the following prescribers on NHS prescription forms?

1 nabilone capsules issued by an independent optometrist prescriber
2 oxycodone hydrochloride capsules issued by an independent nurse prescriber for use in palliative care
3 *Nova-T 380* IUD issued by a community practitioner nurse prescriber

*The answers for this section are on pp. 149–156.*

## CLASSIFICATION QUESTIONS

In this section, for each numbered question, select the one lettered option that most closely corresponds to the answer. Within each group of questions each lettered option may be used once, more than once or not at all.

Questions 1–5 concern the following drugs:

A   digoxin
B   bumetanide
C   lisinopril
D   amiodarone
E   spironolactone

Which of the above:

1   may cause corneal microdeposits?
2   is an aldosterone antagonist?
3   may cause hypokalaemia?
4   may require therapeutic drug monitoring?
5   may cause gynaecomastia?

Questions 6–10 concern the following prescription charges:

A   0
B   1
C   2
D   3
E   4

How many NHS prescription charges do the following items levy (assuming the patient is not exempt for NHS charges)?

6    *Dianette* for acne
7    compression hosiery 2 pairs
8    *Yasmin* oral contraceptive pill
9    warfarin 1 tablet and warfarin 5 mg tablets
10   amoxicillin 500 mg capsule and amoxicillin 250 mg/5 mL syrup

Questions 11–15 concern the following drugs

    A   ciprofloxacin
    B   tramadol
    C   metformin
    D   prednisolone
    E   warfarin

Which of the above:

**11**    may decrease the seizure threshold and cause convulsions?
**12**    may cause glaucoma as a side-effect?
**13**    may cause adrenal suppression?
**14**    may cause drowsiness?
**15**    may cause vitamin $B_{12}$ deficiency?

Questions 16–25 relate to the following controlled drugs:

    A   morphine
    B   temazepam
    C   phenobarbital
    D   diazepam
    E   codeine

Which of the above:

**16**    is a schedule 5 controlled drug?
**17**    is a schedule 2 controlled drug?
**18**    is a schedule 3 controlled drug and may be given as an emergency supply?
**19**    is a schedule 4 controlled drug?
**20**    is a schedule 3 controlled drug and does not require the controlled drug prescription requirements when prescribing?
**21**    has a maximum daily dose of 240 mg?
**22**    may be prescribed for the withdrawal of alcohol?
**23**    is a benzodiazepine and a schedule 3 controlled drug?
**24**    is classed as a strong opioid analgesic?
**25**    is classed as a weak opioid analgesic?

Questions 26–35 concern the following cautionary and advisory labels:

A  Warning. May cause drowsiness. If affected, do not drive or operate machinery. Avoid alcoholic drink

B  May colour the urine

C  Warning. Avoid alcoholic drink

D  Do not stop taking this unless advised by your doctor

E  ... with or after food

Match the cautionary and advisory label with the drug:

26    atenolol tablets
27    ibuprofen tablets
28    metronizadole tablets
29    co-danthramer suspension
30    morphine tablets
31    naproxen tablets
32    amitriptyline tablets
33    prednisolone tablets
34    codeine tablets
35    methadone liquid

Questions 36–40 concern the following drugs:

A  salbutamol
B  aminophylline
C  lithium
D  carbamazepine
E  paracetamol

Which of the above:

36    is indicated for bipolar disorder?
37    may be used to relieve asthma attacks via inhalation?
38    should *not* be given with co-codamol?
39    is a beta$_2$ agonist?
40    is a cytochrome P-450 autoinducer?

Questions 41–50 concern the following drugs:

A  co-amoxiclav
B  atorvastatin
C  amiodarone
D  omeprazole
E  tramadol

Which of the above:

41  can be used in conjunction with other drugs to eradicate *Helicobacter pylori*?
42  should be avoided in penicillin-allergic patients?
43  may be prescribed for secondary prevention of a myocardial infarction?
44  may cause muscle pain?
45  may be prescribed for prophylaxis of a peptic ulcer?
46  is an antiarrhythmic drug?
47  may cause phototoxicity?
48  has some opioid-like effects?
49  may cause drowsiness?
50  is prescribed for moderate pain?

Questions 51–60 concern the following drugs:

A  insulin
B  erythromycin
C  co-careldopa
D  cyclizine
E  aspirin

Which of the above:

51  is a CYT P-450 enzyme inhibitor?
52  is classed as a macrolide?
53  is used for the treatment of Parkinson's disease?
54  is an antiplatelet drug?
55  contains the dopamine precursor, L-dopa?
56  is indicated for vertigo?
57  inhibits COX-1 enzyme?
58  when prescribed needs regular monitoring of the patient's glycosylated haemoglobin?
59  may cause hypoglycaemia as a side-effect?
60  is only available as a parenteral preparation?

Questions 61–70 concern the following drugs:

A  lithium
B  salmeterol
C  methotrexate
D  losartan
E  lactulose

Which of the above:

61    is an osmotic laxative?
62    requires therapeutic drug monitoring?
63    has a similar efficacy to ACE inhibitors but is less likely to cause the dry cough side-effects?
64    may cause pulmonary toxicity?
65    should be given as a weekly dose normally?
66    can be used for hepatic encephalopathy?
67    is a beta$_2$ agonist?
68    may cause nervous tension as a side-effect?
69    is prescribed for mania?
70    is prescribed for bipolar disorder?

Questions 71–73 concern the following herbal remedies:

A    St John's wort
B    green tea
C    echinacea
D    gingko
E    feverfew

Which of the above is traditionally used:

71    for fever?
72    to improve memory?
73    for mild depression?

Questions 74–76 concern the following types of anaemia:

A    pernicious anaemia
B    sickle-cell anaemia
C    aplastic anaemia
D    Cooley's anaemia
E    iron-deficiency anaemia

Which anaemia:

74    is also known as thalassaemia major?
75    results from vitamin B$_{12}$ deficiency?
76    has crescent-shaped red blood cells?

Questions 77–79 concern the following skin conditions:

A   impetigo
B   acne vulgaris
C   scabies
D   plaque psoriasis
E   rosacea

Which of the above:

77   presents with characteristic small grey-blue burrows usually located in the finger webs?
78   is characterised by inflammatory papules and pustules located on the nose and medial cheeks?
79   appears as a small, itchy red patch around the nose and mouth and develops into vesicles that rupture to form a brown-yellow, sticky crust?

Questions 80 and 81 concern the following controlled drugs:

A   nabilone
B   quinalbarbitone
C   diamorphine
D   diazepam
E   kaolin and morphine mixture

Which of the above:

80   does *not* need the prescription to state the dose but, under the Misuse of Drugs Regulations, the prescription has a 28-day validity?
81   does *not* require a licence for import or export?

Questions 82–84 concern the following over-the-counter products:

A   saline nasal drops
B   pseudoephedrine 120 mg tablets
C   acrivastine 8 mg capsule
D   promethazine hydrochloride 10 mg tablets
E   beclometasone dipropionate 0.05% nasal spray

Which of the above:

82    is a sedating antihistamine?
83    requires the patient to seek medical advice if symptoms have not
      improved after 7 days of treatment?
84    can be legally sold in quantities of up to 6 tablets per pack and one pack
      per purchase?

Questions 85–87 concern the following drugs:

A    digoxin
B    lithium
C    phenytoin
D    theophylline
E    ciprofloxacin

Which of the above:

85    has non-linear pharmacokinetics?
86    is cautioned in patients with coeliac disease?
87    is an undesirable choice for teenagers due to its side-effects – coarse
      facies, hirsutism, acne, gingival hyperplasia?

Questions 88 and 89 concern the following drugs:

A    chloroquine base 310 mg o.d.
B    methotrexate tablets 2.5 mg once weekly
C    tamoxifen 20 mg o.d.
D    finasteride 5 mg tablets o.d.
E    lactulose 50 mL t.d.s.

Which of the above:

88    unlicensed for use in women
89    a toxic overdose

Questions 90 and 91 concern different examples of laxatives:

A    This laxative should be carefully swallowed with water and should
      *not* be taken immediately before going to bed
B    In adults, this laxative is usually taken at night, acts in 8–12 hours
      and should be *avoided* in intestinal obstruction
C    This laxative exerts a mild irritant effect and can cause a bowel
      movement in 20 minutes
D    This laxative may also be used in hepatic encephalopathy due to its
      bacteriostatic properties
E    This laxative is used to treat opioid-induced constipation in patients
      receiving palliative care, when response to other laxatives is inadequate

Which of the above statements corresponds to the following drugs?

90    sterculia granules
91    glycerol suppositories

Questions 92 and 93 concern the adverse effects of the following drugs:

A    heparin
B    ciprofloxacin
C    cimetidine
D    lithium
E    digoxin

Which of the above:

92    is cautioned in patients with G6PD deficiency?
93    in toxic doses, may cause the person to have speech difficulties?

Questions 94 and 95 concern the adverse effects of the following drugs:

A    chloroquine phosphate 250 mg tablets
B    clonidine 100 microgram tablets
C    codeine phosphate 60 mg tablets
D    co-codaprin dispersible tablets
E    co-trimoxazole 480 mg tablets

Which of the above drugs carries the following cautionary label:

94    do not take more than 4 in 24 hours?
95    do not stop taking this medicine except on your doctor's advice?

*The answers for this section are on pp. 157–164.*

## STATEMENT QUESTIONS

The questions in this section consist of a statement in the top row followed by a second statement beneath.

You need to:

decide whether the **first** statement is true or false
decide whether the **second** statement is true or false
Then choose:

A     if both statements are true and the second statement is **a correct explanation** of the first statement
B     if both statements are true but the second statement is **NOT a correct explanation** of the first statement
C     if the first statement is true but the second statement is false
D     if the first statement is false but the second statement is true
E     if both statements are false

1     **Statement 1**

Furosemide interacts with lithium

**Statement 2**

Diuretics increase the excretion of lithium

2     **Statement 1**

Methotrexate can be prescribed for rheumatoid arthritis

**Statement 2**

Methotrexate may cause agranulocytosis

3     **Statement 1**

Warfarin is indicated for prophylaxis of deep-vein thrombosis

**Statement 2**

Warfarin is an anticoagulant

4    **Statement 1**

Metformin is first-line antidiabetic therapy for type 2 diabetics with obesity

**Statement 2**

Metformin causes anorexia as a side-effect

5    **Statement 1**

Warfarin interacts with ibuprofen

**Statement 2**

The type of interaction is a pharmacokinetic interaction due to protein binding

6    **Statement 1**

Amiodarone is a drug with a narrow therapeutic range

**Statement 2**

The desired plasma concentration range is 10–20 mg/L

7    **Statement 1**

Temazepam needs to be stored in a controlled drug cupboard

**Statement 2**

Temazepam is a schedule 2 controlled drug

8    **Statement 1**

Parkinson's disease occurs when there is a deficiency of the neurotransmitter dopamine

**Statement 2**

Dopamine does not cross the blood–brain barrier

9 **Statement 1**

Digoxin and bumetanide interact with each other

**Statement 2**

The patient may experience severe hypotension

10 **Statement 1**

Clindamycin is active against Gram-positive cocci and is a broad-spectrum antibiotic

**Statement 2**

Antibiotic-induced colitis may occur with clindamycin

11 **Statement 1**

Enalapril is a beta-blocker

**Statement 2**

Enalapril may cause severe first-dose hypotension

12 **Statement 1**

Phenytoin is indicated for the treatment of epilepsy

**Statement 2**

Phenytoin may cause acne as an adverse effect

13 **Statement 1**

Nabilone is a cannabinoid

**Statement 2**

Nabilone is a schedule 1 controlled drug

14 **Statement 1**

Paroxetine is an antidepressant drug

**Statement 2**

Paroxetine may cause hyponatraemia

15 **Statement 1**

Atenolol is a beta$_2$ adrenoceptor antagonist

**Statement 2**

Atenolol reduces the heart rate

16 **Statement 1**

Patients on regular morphine are also prescribed an antiemetic

**Statement 2**

Morphine may cause nausea and vomiting

17 **Statement 1**

Tramadol has opioid-like effects

**Statement 2**

Tramadol may cause constipation

18 **Statement 1**

Amoxicillin interacts with the combined oral contraceptive pill

**Statement 2**

Patients should be advised to use the barrier method during treatment and for 7 days after stopping antibiotic therapy

19 The 92/27/EEC directive specifies that:

**Statement 1**

All medications supplied must contain their corresponding SPC

**Statement 2**

All medications must be prescribed generically

20 With regard to the following prescription:

Microgynon 30 tablets

1 tablet daily for 21 days; subsequent courses repeated after 7-day tablet-free interval

Mitte 1 OP

**First statement**

A pharmacist can refuse to dispense the above medication based on religious beliefs. However, he or she must refer the patient to another pharmacy which supplies *Microgynon 30*

**Second statement**

Pharmacists who cannot provide a professional service due to religious beliefs are required to notify their employers

21 **First statement**

An audit involves evaluating existing services against set standards

**Second statement**

Community pharmacies are required to complete at least two clinical audits annually, one practice-based audit and one set by the General Pharmaceutical Council

22 Regarding the supply of medical devices in community pharmacy:

**First statement**

Examples of medical devices sold in community pharmacies include blood pressure monitors, contact lenses and condoms

**Second statement**

All medical devices must be marked with CE to show that they have complied with MHRA regulations and to indicate that they are suitable for their intended use with associated risks reduced as far as possible

23 **First statement**

Homeopathic products are the same as herbal products

**Second statement**

The MHRA licenses homeopathic products which may be sold from pharmacies

24 With regard to the following scenario:

Mr X has been coming to your pharmacy to pick up his antidepressants for the past 3 months. He is due to pick up his medicine this week but doesn't show up. One morning he comes into the pharmacy looking thinner and paler than usual.

**First statement**

Symptoms of sudden withdrawal from antidepressants include nausea, vomiting, anorexia and insomnia

**Second statement**

When stopping antidepressants, the dose should be gradually reduced

25 With regard to the following scenario:

On Monday morning, Mrs H, a 49-year-old regular customer, gives you her prescription and asks you if she needs to obtain a formal letter from her doctor as she is travelling with 4 months' supply of nitrazepam. Her prescription reads:

Nitrazepam 5 mg tablets

Take ONE at night

Mitte 112

**First statement**

Nitrazepam is a schedule 4 part II controlled drug

**Second statement**

As Mrs H is travelling with more than 3 months' supply of nitrazepam, she will need to apply for a personal import/export licence from the Home Office before she travels

*The answers for this section are on pp. 165–167.*

# Closed book answers

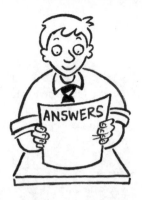

## SIMPLE COMPLETION ANSWERS

**1 A**
Enalapril is an ACE inhibitor and can cause profound first-dose hypotension, therefore it should be initiated at bedtime. See BNF, Chapter 2 (Cardiovascular system), section 2.5.5.1, Angiotensin-converting enzyme inhibitors.

**2 D**
Orlistat is used as an adjunct inobesity. See BNF, Chapter 4 (Central nervous system), section 4.5.1, Anti-obesity drugs acting on the gastro-intestinal tract.

**3 B**
Codeine is a weak opioid. See BNF, Chapter 4 (Central nervous system), section 4.7.2, Opioid analgesics.

**4 A**
Blurred vision is an antimuscarinic side-effect which occurs with all antihistamines, especially the older ones. See BNF, Chapter 3 (Respiratory system), section 3.4.1, Antihistamines.

**5 C**
See BNF, Chapter 2 (Cardiovascular system), section 2.5.5, Drugs affecting the renin–angiotensin system, Heart failure.

**6 C**
Rifampicin colours the urine orange-red.

**7 C**
*Dianette* OC = no charge as contraceptive
Hosiery: 1 charge per stocking = 2 charges
Naproxen = 1 charge
Total = 3 charges

**8 D**
Hypokalaemia (low potassium) predisposes to digoxin toxicity. See BNF, Chapter 2 (Cardiovascular system), section 2.1.1, Cardiac glycosides.

**9 D**
Urinary retention is not a side-effect of beta-blockers. See BNF, Chapter 2 (Cardiovascular system), section 2.4, Beta-adrenoceptor blocking drugs.

**10 E**
Beta-blockers may cause bronchospasm. Therefore, the CSM has advised that beta-blockers should not be given to patients with a history of asthma or bronchospasm. See BNF, Chapter 2 (Cardiovascular system), section 2.4, Beta-adrenoceptor blocking drugs.

**11 D**
Nystagmus is not a side-effect of tricyclic antidepressants. See BNF, Chapter 4 (Central nervous system), section 4.3.1, Tricyclic and related antidepressant drugs.

**12 E**
BMI ranges:

<20 = underweight
20–25 = desired range
25–30 = overweight
>30 = obese

**13 A**
It is advised that diuretics are taken in the morning to minimise inconvenience to the patient visiting the toilet later on in the day.

**14 C**
All are side-effects of GTN, apart from sleep disturbance. See BNF, Chapter 2 (Cardiovascular system), section 2.6.1, Nitrates.

**15 C**
Antimuscarinic side-effects include dry mouth, blurred vision, urinary retention and tachycardia. See BNF, Chapter 4 (Central nervous system), section 4.9.2, Antimuscarinic drugs used in parkinsonism.

**16 A**
All are signs/symptoms of digoxin toxicity except dry mouth. See BNF, Chapter 2 (Cardiovascular system), section 2.1.1, Cardiac glycosides.

**17 D**
Warfarin is an anticoagulant and is indicated for prophylaxis of embolism in atrial fibrillation. See BNF, Chapter 2 (Cardiovascular system), section 2.8.2, Oral anticoagulants.

**18 A**
Doxycycline should be taken with plenty of water. See BNF, Appendix 9, Cautionary and advisory labels for dispensed medicines.

**19 C**
Depot antipsychotics are administered every 1–4 weeks via deep intramuscular injection. See BNF, Chapter 4 (Central nervous system), section 4.2.2, Antipsychotic depot injections.

**20 C**
Women should report any increase in headache frequency or onset of focal symptoms. See BNF, Chapter 7 (Obstetrics, gynaecology, and urinary-tract disorders), section 7.3.1, Combined hormonal contraceptives.

**21 A**
Flucloxacillin's absorption is affected if food is present in the stomach. As a result it should be taken an hour after food or on an empty stomach. See BNF, Appendix 9, Cautionary and advisory labels for dispensed medicines.

**22 B**
Folic acid 400 micrograms daily is advised for women planning a pregnancy. See BNF, Chapter 9 (Nutrition and blood), section 9.1.2, Drugs used in megaloblastic anaemias.

**23 D**
See BNF, Chapter 5 (Infections), section 5.1.9, Antituberculosis drugs.

**24 B**
Amiodarone causes phototoxicity. See BNF, Chapter 2 (Cardiovascular system), section 2.3.2, Drugs for arrhythmias.

**25 A**
There is a possible increased risk of convulsions when quinolones are given with NSAIDs. See BNF, Appendix 1, Interactions.

**26 D**
m/r = Modified-release tablets. These should be swallowed whole and not chewed. See BNF, Appendix 9, Cautionary and advisory labels for dispensed medicines.

**27 E**
Grapefruit juice increases the plasma concentration of simvastatin. See BNF, Appendix 1, Interactions.

**28 B**

**29 C**

**30 D**
'Store in a cool place' requires storage between 8 and 15°C.

**31 D**
The strength of the drug is missing; as more than one strength of atorvastatin is available, the strength must be indicated. For full prescription requirements, see MEP, Section 1.2.3, Prescription-only medicines, Prescriptions for prescription-only medicines.

**32 E**
The doctor's address is missing. For full prescription requirements, see MEP, Section 1.2.3, Prescription-only medicines, Prescriptions for prescription-only medicines.

**33 A**
*Micronor* is an oral contraceptive pill. There is no NHS prescription charge for contraception.

**34 D**
This prescription would be dispensed 4 times (3 repeats + 1st time dispensed = 4). For full prescription requirements, see MEP, Section 1.2.3, Prescription-only medicines, Prescriptions for prescription-only medicines.

**35 D**
Number of days' treatment of lansoprazole is 28, as stated on the prescription. The doctor wishes the patient to take the capsules twice a day (o.m. = in the morning and o.n. = at night). Therefore, 28 days × twice a day = 56.

**36 B**
The address of the doctor is not required on the dispensed label. See MEP, Section 1.2.3, Prescription-only medicines, Emergency supplies of prescription-only medicines.

**37 E**
For emergency supply of the contraceptive pill, a quantity sufficient for a full treatment cycle may be sold or supplied. See MEP, Section 1.2.3, Prescription-only medicines, Emergency supplies of prescription-only medicines.

**38 C**
CD prescriptions are valid for 28 days, not 13 weeks. See MEP, Section 1.2.14, Controlled drugs, Table A: Summary of legal requirements for controlled drugs as they apply to pharmacists.

**39 A**
Temazepam is a schedule 3 CD. See MEP, Section 1.2.14, Controlled drugs, Table A: Summary of legal requirements for controlled drugs as they apply to pharmacists.

**40 B**
The pharmacist needs to record whether the person collecting is the patient, a representative or a healthcare professional. See MEP, Section 1.2.14, Controlled drugs, Table C: Requirements for record keeping of controlled drugs.

**41 B**
Sotalol is a beta-blocker.

**42 D**
Losartan may not cause a dry cough. It is an angiotensin II receptor antagonist and does not cause the degradation of bradykinin, which causes the dry cough with ACE inhibitors.

**43 A**
All may cause hypokalaemia except spironalactone, as it is a potassium-sparing diuretic.

**44 C**
Spinach is very rich in vitamin K.

**45 C**
Clopidogrel is classed as an antiplatelet drug.

**46 A**
Ciclosporin is a narrow therapeutic index drug and requires therapeutic dose monitoring. See BNF, Chapter 8 (Malignant disease and immunosuppression), Section 8.2.2, Corticosteroids and other immunosuppressants.

**47 B**
Salbutamol is a beta$_2$ agonist and has the side-effect of fine tremor.

**48 C**
Naproxen should be taken with or after food to minimise significant gastrointestinal upset.

**49 B**
Metformin is used first-line in type 2 diabetes for obese patients. See BNF, Chapter 6 (Endocrine system), section 6.1.2, Antidiabetic drugs.

**50 B**
Ototoxicity is a toxic effect of gentamicin. See BNF, Chapter 5 (Infections), section 5.1.4, Aminoglycosides.

**51 A**
A preterm baby is defined as less than 37 weeks' gestational age.

**52 E**
Pyrexia is defined as a body temperature of greater than 37.5°C (99.5°F) in children under the age of 5 and 38°C (100.4°F) or over in those aged 5 or over. See NHS guidelines on fever (available online at: www.nhs.uk/chq/Pages/1633. aspx?CategoryID=62&SubCategoryID=64.

**53 E**
Troch. is the Latin abbreviation for *trochisci* which means lozenges.

**54 D**
See BNF, Chapter 12 (Ear, nose, and oropharynx), section 12.3.1, Drugs for oral ulceration and inflammation, Corticosteroids.

**55 E**
Traditional uses of Asian ginseng include boosting the immune system and improving both mental and physical performance.

**56 D**
The priority in acute diarrhoea is to prevent or reverse fluid and electrolyte depletion. See BNF, Chapter 1 (Gastro-intestinal system), section 1.4, Acute diarrhoea.

**57 A**

**58 B**

**59 D**
See MEP 33, Chapter 3, Improving pharmacy practice, Section 3.2, Practice guidance documents, Substances of misuse.

**60 C**
See MEP, Section 1.2.3, Prescription-only medicines (POM), Emergency supplies of prescription-only medicines.

**61 D**
Methadone is a schedule 2 controlled drug which is used to treat opioid misusers and can only be legally prescribed and dispensed against a valid instalment prescription. Pharmacists must be aware of the abuse potential of any controlled drug. See MEP, Section 1.2.14, Controlled drugs, National Health prescriptions for the treatment of misusers.

**62 C**
Repeat dispensing is an essential service. MURs and Prescription Intervention Service is an advanced service and the remaining services are all enhanced services. See the NHS contract.

**63 D**
Storing or destroying industrial waste, e.g. medicinal waste from doctors or nursing homes, requires a licence from the Environmental Agency. See MEP, Section 1.2.13, Handling of waste medicines.

**64 A**
All CD POMs (schedule 2 CDs) which are pharmacy stock require an authorised witness to be present for their destruction. Benzfetamine (minor stimulant) is CD no reg. POM, and therefore does not need an authorised witness. All the remaining stock are CD POMs. See MEP, Section 1.2.14, Controlled drugs, Schedule 2 drugs; RPSGB *Law and Ethics Bulletin*, New additions to the list of controlled drugs; Destruction of controlled drugs.

**65 C**
See MEP 33, Chapter 3, Improving pharmacy practice, Section 3.2, Practice guidance documents, Emergency hormonal contraception.

**66 E**
A separate room with a separate sink should be used for the pregnancy test. See MEP 33, Chapter 3, Improving pharmacy practice, Section 3.2, Practice guidance documents, Pregnancy testing in the pharmacy.

**67 B**
See MEP 33, Chapter 3, Improving pharmacy practice, Section 3.2, Practice guidance documents, Medical devices.

**68 B**
See MEP 33, Chapter 3, Improving pharmacy practice, Section 3.2, Practice guidance documents, Counterfeit medicines.

**69 A**
See MEP, Section 1.2.14, Controlled drugs, Supplying drug paraphernalia; MEP 33, Chapter 3, Improving pharmacy practice, Section 3.2, Practice guidance documents, Best practice guidance for commissioners and providers of pharmaceutical services for drug users.

**70 E**
The CE (*conformité européenne*) mark is marked on certain products that meet the safety standards that apply to all countries of the European Union. For more information, see MEP 33, Chapter 3, Improving pharmacy practice, Section 3.2, Practice guidance documents, Medical devices.

**71 D**
Misoprostol. See individual monographs in the BNF.

**72 B**
Phenothiazines. See BNF, Chapter 4 (Central nervous system), section 4.2.1, Antipsychotic drugs, Side-effects.

**73 B**
Digoxin is *not* hepatotoxic. Refer to individual monographs in the BNF.

**74 C**
Refer to relevant Responding to Symptoms textbook and BNF, Chapter 5 (Infections), section 5.4.1, Antimalarials, Prophylaxis against malaria.

**75 E**
The cause of migraine has been associated with low serotonin levels, hormonal changes and some drugs, e.g. bupropion.

**76 E**
A common side-effect of quinolones is diarrhoea. See separate BNF entries.

**77 B**

**78 B**
Clioquinol is present in some topical applications and can stain skin and clothes. The colour effects of the remaining drugs are as follows: triamterene: urine may look slightly blue in some lights; levodopa: occasionally, dark colour, i.e. red, brown or black, may appear in saliva, urine or sweat; co-danthramer: red urine; rifampicin: red-orange colour in the urine, sweat and tears.

**79 D**
The storage conditions for *Humulin M3* pen 100 IU/mL suspension for injection are as follows: before first use the pen is to be stored in a refrigerator (2–8°C). When used, the pen is to be stored at room temperature (below 30°C) for up to 28 days. Do not keep your 'in use' pen in the fridge. Do not put it near heat or in the sun and do not freeze. See PIL for *Humulin M3* pen.

**80 E**
Phenytoin. See individual monographs in the BNF.

**81 C**
See individual monographs in the BNF, and see MEP 33, Chapter 3, Improving pharmacy practice, Section 3.2, Practice guidance documents, Hazardous Waste (England and Wales) Regulations 2005, Interim guidance for community pharmacists, List of 'hazardous' medicines.

**82 C**
A is under the licensed age (45–75 years) and needs to be referred as he may have diabetes. B needs to be referred as his symptoms point to kidney disease. For D, concomitant use of any other alpha$_1$-blocker is contraindicated. E: not licensed for use in women. See MEP 33, Chapter 3, Improving pharmacy practice, Section 3.2, Practice guidance documents, (OTC tamsulosin). See http://www.rpharms.com/practice–science-and-research/otc-tamsulosin-reference-guide.asp.

**83 E**
NHS near the name of the drug means that the preparation in question cannot be prescribed on the NHS, i.e. it is blacklisted. Refer to recent *Drug Tariff* for up-to-date list. See BNF, How to use the BNF.

**84 E**
Treatment depends on symptoms, extent of overdose and length of time for the overdose. In acute overdose treatment may be supportive with special regard to electrolyte balance, renal function and control of convulsions. See BNF, Emergency treatment of poisoning, Specific drugs, Lithium.

**85 C**
Visual disturbances, such as objects appearing yellow or green, are a sign of digoxin toxicity.

**86 E**
*Alli* can only be sold to a person with a BMI of 28 kg/m$^2$ or higher. See MEP 33, Chapter 3, Improving pharmacy practice, Section 3.2, Practice guidance documents, Orlistat.

**87 D**
Ketoconazole is contraindicated in active liver disease. See BNF, Chapter 5 (Infections), section 5.2.2, Imidazole antifungals, Ketoconazole.

**88 D**
Ringworm is a fungal infection which may be contracted from infected animals or people. It starts as a red spot which spreads outwards to form an inflamed 'ring'.

**89 D**
Allopurinol should not be taken during an acute gout attack as it may prolong the attack indefinitely. See BNF, Chapter 10 (Musculoskeletal and joint diseases), section 10.1.4, Gout and cytotoxic-induced hyperuricaemia, Acute attacks of gout.

**90 E**
See BNF, Emergency treatment of poisoning, Specific drugs, Stimulants, Cocaine.

**91 C**
See BNF, Appendix 1, Interactions, List of drug interactions, Aspirin.

**92 E**
The brand should be specified for all the listed drugs except digoxin due to the variations in properties of the different available formulations. See individual BNF entries.

**93 E**
Side-effects of drugs which affect the patient's ability to drive or operate machinery safely include drowsiness, dizziness, blurred vision (or visual disturbances) and nausea. All central nervous system depressants or antihistamines (both sedating and non-sedating) may cause drowsiness. $\alpha_1$-blockers may cause syncope, dizziness or blurred vision. See individual BNF entries and Appendix 9, Cautionary and advisory labels for dispensed medicines, Recommended label wordings, 1, 2 and 3.

**94 B**
See NHS advice on drinking limits.

**95 D**
Symptoms of liver disease may include anorexia, nausea, vomiting, fatigue, abdominal pain (upper right region), jaundice or dark urine.

**96 D**

Colestyramine is a bile acid sequestrant which can interfere with the absorption of fat-soluble vitamins, i.e. vitamins A, D, E and K. Patients who are taking other drugs should be advised to take them at least 1 hour before or 4–6 hours after bile acid sequestrants to reduce possible interference with absorption. See BNF, Chapter 2 (Cardiovascular system), section 2.12, Lipid-regulating drugs, Bile acid sequestrants.

**97 E**

Prolonged use of the topical sympathomimetics can lead to rebound congestion (rhinitis medicamentosa).

**98 A**

Pharmacists are expected to know the exemptions for NHS prescription payment. All NHS prescriptions are free in Wales. See *Drug Tariff*, Part XVI, Notes on charges.

**99 E**

Medical devices sold in a pharmacy may include needles, syringes, dressings, thermometers, blood pressure monitors, stoma care products, glucose meters, test strips, inhalers, condoms, test kits, e.g. cholesterol, pregnancy, screening tests, e.g. PSA, faecal blood. See MEP 33, Chapter 3, Improving pharmacy practice, Section 3.2, Practice guidance documents, Medical devices.

**100 E**

The Department of Health has stated that appliances will not be eligible for entry into the list of drugs for which discount is not deducted. See *Drug Tariff*, Part II and PSNC website for further details.

**101 E**

Minoxidil solution for external use is a 'black list' item which cannot be prescribed on the NHS. See *Drug Tariff*, Parts XVIIIA and XVIIIB.

**102 C**

Although these are the same brands for carbamazepine, they are two different formulations. See *Drug Tariff*, Part XVI, Notes on charges, Notes on the number of charges payable.

**103 C**

Cyproterone acetate with ethinylestradiol (co-cyprindiol or *Dianette*) contains an antiandrogen and thus may be used for severe acne or moderately severe hirsutism. See BNF, Chapter 13 (Skin), section 13.6.2, Oral preparations for acne, Hormone treatment for acne.

## MULTIPLE COMPLETION ANSWERS

**1 A**
Pharmacodynamic interactions are interactions between drugs that have similar or antagonistic pharmacological effects. See BNF, Appendix 1, Interactions.

**2 D**
Pharmacokinetic interactions occur when a drug alters the absorption, metabolism, distribution or excretion of another drug, which in turn reduces or increases its pharmacological effects. See BNF, Appendix 1, Interactions.

**3 C**
Taste disturbance and black stools are not side-effects of insulin. See BNF, Chapter 6 (Endocrine system), section 6.1.1, Insulin.

**4 A**
Migraines, abdominal cramps and liver impairment are side-effects of combined oral contraceptive pills, such as *Yasmin*. See BNF, Chapter 7 (Obstetrics, gynaecology, and urinary-tract disorders), section 7.3.1, Combined hormonal contraceptives.

**5 E**
Levothyroxine is the only one on the list indicated for hypothyroidism. See BNF, Chapter 6 (Endocrine system), section 6.2.1, Thyroid hormones.

**6 B**
Malathion liquid is indicated for head lice and crab lice but not for threadworm.

**7 A**
Mrs Naqvi may experience osteoporosis, glaucoma and/or diabetes. These are all side-effects of glucocorticoid therapy. See BNF, Chapter 6 (Endocrine system), section 6.3.2, Glucocorticoid therapy.

**8 B**
Fludrocortisone has glucorticoid activity; however its mineralocorticoid effects are more potent – 100 times greater than hydrocortisone. See BNF, Chapter 6 (Endocrine system), section 6.3, Corticosteroids.

**9 A**

All three parameters need to be regularly monitored in diabetic patients. See BNF, Chapter 6 (Endocrine system), section 6.1, Drugs used in diabetes.

**10 E**

Glycosylated haemoglobin demonstrates long-term glycaemic control. See BNF, Chapter 6 (Endocrine system), section 6.1, Drugs used in diabetes.

**11 A**

All three are used for the prophylaxis of malaria. See BNF, Chapter 5 (Infections), section 5.4.1, Antimalarials.

**12 B**

Nystatin is a POM and cannot be counter-prescribed as it is not indicated for vaginal candidiasis. *Diflucan One* and *Canesten* pessaries are classified as P and can be prescribed over the counter.

**13 C**

Metronidazole is not indicated for UTIs. Trimethroprim and nitrofurantoin are indicated for UTIs. See BNF, Chapter 5 (Infections), section 5.1.13, Urinary-tract infections.

**14 B**

Toxic effects of vancomycin include nephrotoxicity and ototoxicity. See BNF, Chapter 5 (Infections), section 5.1.7, Some other antibacterials.

**15 A**

All three are correct. See BNF, Chapter 5 (Infections), section 5.1.3, Tetracyclines.

**16 D**

Only gabapentin is indicated for neuropathic pain.

**17 B**

Morphine is classed as a strong opioid and it may cause respiratory depression. It is a schedule 2 CD. See BNF, Chapter 4 (Central nervous system), section 4.7.2, Opioid analgesics.

**18 D**

Acarbose is indicated for diabetes. Glucagon and diazoxide are indicated for hypoglycaemia and chronic hypoglycaemia respectively. See BNF, Chapter 6 (Endocrine system), section 6.1.4, Treatment of hypoglycaemia.

**19 E**
The prescription must be sent to the pharmacy in 72 hours. The prescription-only medicine cannot be a schedule 1, 2 or 3 controlled drug. See MEP, Section 1.2.3, Prescription-only medicines, Emergency supplies of prescription-only medicines.

**20 A**
All three are correct. See MEP, Section 1.2.3, Prescription-only medicines, Pharmacist prescribers.

**21 A**
All three are correct. See MEP, Section 1.2.3, Prescription-only medicines, Patient group directions.

**22 C**
See MEP, Section 1.2.3, Prescription-only medicines, Facsimile transmission of prescriptions.

**23 B**
A dentist *can* make an emergency supply request. See MEP, Section 1.2.3, Prescription-only medicines, Validity of dental prescriptions.

**24 E**
Paracetamol and ibuprofen, sold in a quantity of 16, are classed as GSL items. Ranitidine is a P medicine. See MEP, Section 1.3, Alphabetical list of medicines for human use.

**25 A**
All three are GSL products. See MEP, Section 1.3, Alphabetical list of medicines for human use.

**26 D**
GTN tablets are a P item and *Oilatum* gel is a GSL item. See MEP, Section 1.3, Alphabetical list of medicines for human use.

**27 B**
Paracetamol tablets – if the quantity is greater than 32 – are classed as a POM item. *Ovex* tablets (for threadworm) are classed as a P item. See MEP, Section 1.3, Alphabetical list of medicines for human use.

**28 A**
See MEP, Section 1.3, Alphabetical list of medicines for human use.

**29 A**
See MEP, Section 1.3, Alphabetical list of medicines for human use.

**30 B**
Diltiazem and bumetanide is not a black dot interaction; however, they do interact and may enhance the hypotensive effect. This is something that can be monitored. See BNF, Appendix 1, Interactions.

**31 A**
Bleeding from any orifice is an alarm feature for immediate referral.

**32 A**

**33 B**

**34 D**
See MEP 33, Chapter 3, Improving pharmacy practice, Section 3.2, Practice guidance documents, Standards checklist for registered pharmacy premises.

**35 A**
See MEP, Section 1.2.3, Prescription-only medicines (POM), Forged prescriptions, and MEP 33, Chapter 3, Improving pharmacy practice, Section 3.2, Practice guidance documents, Substances of misuse.

**36 C**
See MEP, Section 3.1, Continuing professional development.

**37 D**
See MEP, Section 1.2.14, Controlled drugs, Prescriptions for controlled drugs; Destruction of controlled drugs, Obsolete, expired and unwanted stock controlled drugs, or Methods and procedures; National Health prescriptions for the treatment of misusers.

**38 B**
See MEP, Section 1.2.14, Controlled drugs, Prescriptions for controlled drugs, and Repeat prescription; Prescribing for up to 30 days' clinical need; Table A: Summary of legal requirements for controlled drugs or corresponding schedule monographs.

**39 A**
See MEP 33, Section 3.1.1, Clinical governance.

**40 B**
Any circumstances which affect the pharmacist's fitness to practise or may bring the profession into disrepute, e.g. ill health or criminal convictions, must be reported to the General Pharmaceutical Council. See http://www.pharmacyregulation.org/aboutus/whoweare/committees/statutorycommittees/fitnesstopracticecommittee/index.aspx.

**41 B**
The description of statement 3 is that of continuous professional development. See MEP 33, Section 3.1.1, Clinical governance.

**42 B**
Buprenorphine may be issued by instalments only if it is written on the correct form (in England FP10MDA). Repeat prescriptions for both schedule 2 and 3 are not allowed. See MEP, Section 1.2.14, Controlled drugs, Repeat prescriptions; National Health prescriptions for the treatment of misusers.

**43 D**
MEP 33, Chapter 3, Improving pharmacy practice, Section 3.2, Practice guidance documents, Developing and implementing standard operating procedures for dispensing.

**44 B**
MEP 33, Chapter 3, Improving pharmacy practice, Section 3.2, Practice guidance documents, Child protection.

**45 A**
See MEP 33, Section 2.1, Code of ethics for pharmacists and pharmacy technicians, The seven principles.

**46 B**
Veterinary prescribers are not allowed to request an emergency supply. See MEP, Section 1.2.3, Prescription-only medicines (POM), Emergency supplies of prescription-only medicines.

**47 A**
An unlicensed medicine is defined as a medicinal product which does not have a product licence or marketing authorisation within the UK.

**48 A**
See BNF, Chapter 5 (Infections), section 5.1.11, Metronidazole and tinidazole, and section 1.5, Chronic bowel disorders, *Clostridium difficile* infection.

**49 B**
The third statement is incorrect because it is the short-acting GTN tablets which have a shelf-life of 8 weeks. See separate entries in BNF.

**50 B**
Lipophilic drugs can readily cross cell membranes and hence have a high apparent volume of distribution. These drugs can only be excreted from the body after they have been transformed into more polar compounds by the liver.

**51 A**
See BNF, Chapter 10 (Musculoskeletal and joint diseases), section 10.1.4, Gout and cytotoxic-induced hyperuricaemia, Long-term control of gout, Allopurinol.

**52 B**
Depot injections of conventional antipsychotics may give rise to a higher incidence of extrapyramidal reactions than oral preparations. See BNF, Chapter 4 (Central nervous system), section 4.2.2, Antipsychotic depot injections.

**53 A**
Different formulations of all of the listed drugs have different properties. To avoid confusion and subtherapeutic or adverse effects, prescribers should specify the brand to be dispensed. See individual BNF entries.

**54 A**
See BNF, Chapter 2 (Cardiovascular system), section 2.4, Beta-adrenoceptor blocking drugs.

**55 E**
Pharmacists who receive a script for generically prescribed lithium must first ascertain the previously administered brand with the prescriber as available preparations vary widely in their bioavailabilities. See BNF, Chapter 4 (Central nervous system), section 4.2.3, Antimanic drugs, Lithium.

**56 A**
Patients who are at a higher risk of developing peripheral neuropathy with isoniazid include individuals who have HIV infection, malnutrition, alcohol dependence, diabetes and chronic renal failure. These patients should be given pyridoxine 10 mg daily prophylactically from the start of their treatment. See BNF, Chapter 5 (Infections), section 5.1.9, Antituberculosis drugs, Isoniazid.

**57 C**
The symptoms of the 17-year-old boy are indicative of diabetes mellitus. Any patients over the age of 55 with unexplained, recent-onset dyspepsia which has not responded to treatment should be referred for further investigation.

**58 E**
Ciclosporin should be prescribed and dispensed by brand name due to the clinically important differences in bioavailability between brands. See BNF, Chapter 8 (Malignant disease and immunosuppression), section 8.2.2, Corticosteroids and other immunosuppressants, Ciclosporin.

**59 B**
Persistent dry cough, shortness of breath, sudden weight loss and fever may indicate pneumonitis, a life-threatening adverse effect of amiodarone. Statement 3 is incorrect because if hypothydroidism develops it can be treated with replacement therapy without withdrawing amiodarone. However if amiodarone causes severe hepatic impairment it should be discontinued by a specialist. See BNF, Chapter 2 (Cardiovascular system), section 2.3.2, Drugs for arrhythmias, Supraventricular and ventricular arrhythmias, Amiodarone hydrochloride.

**60 D**
Both verapamil and erythromycin increase serum theophylline levels. See BNF, Appendix 1, Interactions, Theophylline.

**61 B**
Pethidine hydrochloride is a synthetic opioid which, like other opioids, may cause constipation. Other common opioid side-effects are nausea, vomiting, dry mouth and biliary spasm. See separate BNF entries.

**62 D**
*Marvelon* is a combined oral contraceptive which contains desogestrel 150 micrograms and ethinylestradiol 30 micrograms. Griseofulvin is a hepatic enzyme inducer which increases metabolism of oestrogens or progestogens and thus decreases the contraceptive effect of oral combined, oral progestogen-only, patches and vaginal ring contraceptives. Short-term use of enzyme inducers necessitates the use of extra contraceptive measures during treatment and for 4 weeks afterwards. See BNF, Chapter 7 (Obstetrics, gynaecology, and urinary-tract disorders), section 7.3.1, Combined hormonal contraceptives, Interactions.

**63 C**
See BNF, Chapter 5 (Infections), section 5.1, Antibacterial drugs, Table 1, Summary of antibacterial therapy, Urinary tract.

**64 D**
Anaphylactic reactions occur in fewer than 0.05% of treated patients. Individuals with a history of a rash that occurs more than 72 hours after penicillin administration are probably not allergic to penicillin. However, the possibility of an allergic reaction should be borne in mind. See BNF, Chapter 5 (Infections), section 5.1.1, Penicillins, Hypersensitivity reactions.

**65 A**
See BNF, Chapter 4 (Central nervous system), section 4.3.2, Monoamine-oxidase inhibitors, Interactions.

**66 A**
Refer to individual BNF sections.

**67 A**
Aspirin reduces the excretion of methotrexate and thus increases the risk of toxicity. Patients should therefore be advised to avoid self-medication with aspirin or other NSAIDs. Aspirin may cause haemolysis in G6PD-deficient patients. Aspirin or other NSAIDs are contraindicated in patients with a history of hypersensitivity (e.g. hives) to any NSAID or aspirin. See BNF, Chapter 2 (Cardiovascular system), section 2.9, Antiplatelet drugs, Aspirin (antiplatelet); Chapter 9 (Nutrition and blood), section 9.1, Anaemias and some other blood disorders, section 9.1.5, G6PD deficiency, and Chapter 10 (Musculoskeletal and joint diseases), section 10.1.3, Drugs that suppress the rheumatic disease process, Drugs affecting the immune response, Methotrexate.

**68 C**
Optometrist independent prescribers are not allowed to prescribe any controlled drugs. Independent nurse prescribers can prescribe listed CDs (Part XVIIBii of the *Drug Tariff*) for the specified circumstances and community practitioner nurse prescribers can prescribe the listed products in *Drug Tariff*, Parts XVIIBi, IXA, IXB, IXC and IXR except where the (N) symbol appears.

## CLASSIFICATION ANSWERS

**1 D**
Amiodarone may cause corneal microdeposits as an adverse effect.

**2 E**
Spironolactone is an aldosterone antagonist.

**3 B**
Bumetanide is a loop diuretic and may cause hypokalaemia as a side-effect.

**4 A**
Digoxin is a narrow therapeutic index drug and may require therapeutic dose monitoring.

**5 E**
Spironolatone may cause gynaecomastia in males as an adverse effect.

**6 B**
Although *Dianette* is an oral contraceptive pill and may be free of charge, it incurs a charge if prescribed for acne rather than contraception.

**7 E**
With stockings/hosiery, 1 charge applies per piece of hosiery. So 2 pairs = 4 pieces, therefore, 4 charges should be levied.

**8 A**
*Yasmin* is an oral contraceptive pill and is free of charge.

**9 B**
The *same* drug with the *same* formulation, but different strengths, is classed as 1 prescription charge.

**10 C**
The *same* drug, but *different* formulation, is classed as a charge per item, therefore there will be 2 prescription charges.

**11 A**
Ciprofloxacin decreases the seizure threshold and causes convulsions.

**12 D**
Prednisolone is a glucocorticoid and may cause glaucoma as an adverse effect.

**13 D**
Prednisolone may cause adrenal suppression.

**14 B**
Tramadol has opioid-like effects and may cause drowsiness.

**15 C**
Metformin may cause vitamin $B_{12}$ deficiency.

**16 E**
Codeine is a schedule 5 CD.

**17 A**
Morphine is a schedule 2 CD.

**18 C**
Phenobarbital may be given as an emergency supply if it is indicated for epilepsy.

**19 D**
Diazepam is a schedule 4 part I CD.

**20 B**
Prescription of temazepam does not have controlled drug prescription requirements.

**21 E**
The maximum amount of codeine in 24 hours is 240 mg.

**22 D**
Diazepam can be prescribed for the withdrawal of alcohol.

**23 B**
Temazepam and diazepam are both benzodiazepines, but temazepam is a schedule 3 controlled drug, whereas diazepam is a schedule 4 controlled drug.

**24 A**
Morphine is a strong opioid (according to the WHO pain ladder).

**25 E**
Codeine is classed as a weak opioid (according to the WHO pain ladder).
Full explanations for the following answers are given in the BNF, Appendix
9, Cautionary and advisory labels for dispensed medicines.

**26 D**

**27 E**

**28 C**

**29 B**

**30 A**

**31 E**

**32 A**

**33 D**

**34 A**

**35 A**

**36 C**
Lithium is indicated for bipolar disorder.

**37 A**
Salbutamol is the 'reliever' and is used in patients who are having an attack.

**38 E**
Paracetamol should not be given with co-codamol as the latter contains
paracetamol.

**39 A**
Salbutamol is a beta$_2$ agonist.

**40 D**
Carbamazepine is a cytochrome P450 autoinducer.

**41 D**
See BNF, Chapter 1 (Gastro-intestinal system), section 1.3, Antisecretory drugs and mucosal protectants.

**42 A**
See BNF, Chapter 5 (Infections), section 5.1.1, Penicillins.

**43 B**
See BNF, Chapter 2 (Cardiovascular system), section 2.12, Lipid-regulating drugs.

**44 B**
See BNF, Chapter 2 (Cardiovascular system), section 2.12, Lipid-regulating drugs.

**45 D**
See BNF, Chapter 1 (Gastro-intestinal system), section 1.3, Antisecretory drugs and mucosal protectants.

**46 C**
See BNF, Chapter 2 (Cardiovascular system), section 2.3.2, Drugs for arrhythmias.

**47 C**
See BNF, Chapter 2 (Cardiovascular system), section 2.3.2, Drugs for arrhythmias.

**48 E**
See BNF, Chapter 4 (Central nervous system), section 4.7.2, Opioid analgesics.

**49 E**
See BNF, Chapter 4 (Central nervous system), section 4.7.2, Opioid analgesics.

**50 E**
See BNF, Chapter 4 (Central nervous system), section 4.7.2, Opioid analgesics.

**51 B**
Erythromycin is a cytochrome P450 enzyme inhibitor.

**52 B**
Erythromycin is classed as a macrolide.

**53 C**
Co-careldopa is used in the treatment of Parkinson's disease.

**54 E**
Aspirin is an antiplatelet drug.

**55 C**
Co-careldopa contains the dopamine precursor, l-dopa.

**56 D**
See BNF, Chapter 4 (Central nervous system), section 4.6, Drugs used in nausea and vertigo.

**57 E**
Aspirin inhibits COX-1 enzyme.

**58 A**
See BNF, Chapter 6 (Endocrine system), section 6.1.1, Insulins.

**59 A**
See BNF, Chapter 6 (Endocrine system), section 6.1.1, Insulins.

**60 A**
See BNF, Chapter 6 (Endocrine system), section 6.1.1, Insulins.

**61 E**
See BNF, Chapter 1 (Gastro-intestinal system), section 1.6.4, Peripheral opioid-receptor antagonists.

**62 A**
Lithium requires therapeutic drug monitoring.

**63 D**
See BNF, Chapter 2 (Cardiovascular system), section 2.5.5.2, Angiotensin-II receptor antagonists.

**64 C**
See BNF, Chapter 10 (Musculoskeletal and joint diseases), section 10.1.3, Drugs that suppress the rheumatic disease process.

**65 C**
See BNF, Chapter 10 (Musculoskeletal and joint diseases), section 10.1.3, Drugs that suppress the rheumatic disease process.

**66 E**
See BNF, Chapter 1 (Gastro-intestinal system), section 1.6.4, Osmotic laxatives.

**67 B**
See BNF, Chapter 3 (Respiratory system), section 3.1.1, Adrenoceptor agonists.

**68 B**
See BNF, Chapter 3 (Respiratory system), section 3.1.1, Adrenoceptor agonists.

**69 A**

**70 A**
For answers 71–73: these are only common or traditional uses and further studies are required to provide evidence for their clinical effectiveness.

**71 E**

**72 D**

**73 A**

**74 D**

**75 A**

**76 B**

**77 C**

**78 E**

**79 A**

**80 D**
Diazepam is Schedule 4 Part I (CD Benz POM). The only prescription requirement from the Misuse of Drugs Regulations 2001 is the 28-day validity. The other requirements fall under the Medicines Act 1968. See MEP, Section 1.2.14, Controlled drugs, Schedule 4 drugs.

**81 E**
Kaolin and morphine mixture is Schedule 5 (CD Inv) and thus does not require a licence for import or export. See MEP, Section 1.2.14, Controlled drugs, Schedule 5 drugs.

**82 D**
See BNF, Chapter 3 (Respiratory system), section 3.4.1 Antihistamines, Sedating antihistamines.

**83 E**

**84 B**
See MEP, Section 1.2.3, Prescription-only medicines (POM), Exemptions from prescription-only medicine status, Exemptions for products consisting of or containing pseudoephedrine salts or ephedrine base or salts.

**85 C**
See BNF, Chapter 4 (Central nervous system), section 4.8.1, Control of epilepsy, Phenytoin.

**86 E**
Quinolones should be used with caution in patients with a history of epilepsy or conditions that predispose to seizures such as coeliac disease. See BNF, Chapter 5 (Infections), section 5.1.12, Quinolones.

**87 C**
See BNF, Chapter 4 (Central nervous system), section 4.8.1, Control of epilepsy, Phenytoin.

**88 D**
See BNF, Chapter 6 (Endocrine system), section 6.4.2, Male sex hormones and antagonists, Anti-androgens, Dutasteride, Finasteride.

**89 A**
See BNF, Chapter 5 (Infections), section 5.4.1, Antimalarials, Chloroquine, Side-effects.

**90 A**
Preparations that swell in contact with liquid should be carefully swallowed with water and should *not* be taken immediately before going to bed. See BNF, Chapter 1 (Gastro-intestinal system), section 1.6.1, Bulk-forming laxatives.

**91 C**
Glycerol acts by means of a mildly irritating effect to stimulate a bowel movement quickly. See BNF, Chapter 1 (Gastro-intestinal system), section 1.6.2, Stimulant laxatives.

**92 B**

Quinolones antibiotics increase the risk of haemolysis in most G6PD-deficient patients. See BNF, Chapter 9 (Nutrition and blood), section 9.1.5, G6PD deficiency.

**93 D**

Ataxia is a toxic effect of lithium. It is the loss of muscle coordination, e.g. difficulty speaking. Other toxic effects include tremor, dysarthria, nystagmus, renal impairment and convulsions. See BNF, Chapter 4 (Central nervous system), section 4.2.3, Antimanic drugs, Lithium.

**94 C**

Maximum daily dose of codeine phosphate is 240 mg. See BNF, Chapter 4 (Central nervous system), section 4.7.2, Opioid analgesics, Codeine phosphate.

**95 B**

Sudden withdrawal of clonidine may cause hypertensive crises. See BNF, Appendix 9, Cautionary and advisory labels for dispensed medicines.

## STATEMENT ANSWERS

**1 C**
Diuretics decrease the excretion of lithium. See BNF, Appendix 1, Interactions.

**2 B**

**3 A**

**4 A**

**5 C**

**6 E**

**7 C**
Temazepam is a schedule 3 controlled drug.

**8 B**
See BNF, Chapter 4 (Central nervous system), section 4.9, Drugs used in parkinsonism and related disorders.

**9 C**
The explanation of the interaction is incorrect. Bumetanide may cause hypo-kalaemia, which in turn may precipitate digoxin toxicity. See BNF, Appendix 1, Interactions.

**10 A**
Broad-spectrum antibiotics may induce antibiotic-induced colitis due to the short-term eradication of the gut flora. See BNF, Chapter 5 (Infections), section 5.1.6, Clindamycin.

**11 D**
Enalapril is an ACE inhibitor and may cause a profound first-dose hypotension.

**12 B**

**13 C**
Nabilone is not a schedule 1 controlled drug.

**14 B**

**15 B**

**16 A**

**17 A**

**18 B**

**19 E**
The directive specifies that any medication supplied to a patient must contain a patient information leaflet. A Summary of Product Characteristics (SPC) provides more details on the medicines properties. Prescribers are advised to use non-proprietary names (generic) when prescribing. However, this is not always the case, as some preparations may vary in clinical effect between different manufacturers. See 92/27/EEC directive and BNF, Guidance on prescribing, General guidance, Non-proprietary titles.

**20 B**
Pharmacists are permitted to refuse to deliver a service based on religious beliefs; however, they must inform the relevant persons and refer the patient appropriately. See MEP 33, Section 2.1, Code of ethics for pharmacists and pharmacy technicians, 3. Show respect for others.

**21 C**
The second audit will be set by the PCT. See MEP 33, Section 3, Improving pharmacy practice, Audit see http://www.uptodate.org.uk/home/welcome.shtml.

**22 B**
MEP 33, Chapter 3 (Respiratory system), Improving pharmacy practice, Section 3.2, Practice guidance documents, Medical devices.

**23 D**
MEP 33, Chapter 3 (Respiratory system), Improving pharmacy practice, Section 3.2, Practice guidance documents, Homeopathic and herbal products advice for pharmacists.

**24 B**
Antidepressants (particularly MAOIs) which are stopped suddenly after regular administration for 8 weeks or more cause sudden withdrawal symptoms and should therefore be stopped through gradual dose reduction. See BNF, Chapter 4 (Central nervous system), section 4.3, Antidepressant drugs, withdrawal.

**25 D**
Nitrazepam is a CD Benz POM. Travellers who are carrying certain controlled drugs for their own use abroad (or into the UK) in quantities which exceed 3 months' supply (or if the person is travelling for 3 months or more) must obtain a *personal licence* from the Home Office. For any other drugs or for travel periods of less than 3 months, it is advisable to obtain a letter from the prescribing doctor. See BNF, Guidance on prescribing, Controlled Drugs and drug dependence.

# Calculation questions

Naba Elsaid

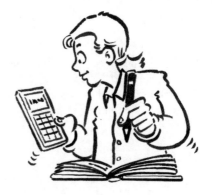

## SIMPLE COMPLETION QUESTIONS

Each of the questions or statements in this section is followed by five suggested answers. Select the best answer in each situation.

1   A formula requires 200 mL of single-strength chloroform water. You have concentrated chloroform water in stock. What volume of this is needed to prepare the required formula?

   A   5 mL
   B   10 mL
   C   100 mL
   D   200 mL
   E   400 mL

2   Mrs T has been stabilised on digoxin tablets 250 micrograms daily. She is no longer able to swallow her tablets and her doctor decides to change her to an equivalent dose of the elixir. Given that the bioavailability of digoxin is 0.65 for the tablets and 0.8 for the elixir, calculate the dose of elixir needed:

   A   0.004 mL
   B   0.04 mL
   C   0.4 mL
   D   4 mL
   E   40 mL

3   What weight of alcometasone dipropionate 0.05% is present in 40 g of *Modrasone* cream?

   A   0.002 mg
   B   0.02 mg
   C   0.2 mg
   D   2 mg
   E   20 mg

4   Mr A has been prescribed enoximone 20 micrograms/kg/min to be administered by continuous intravenous infusion. Given that Mr A weighs 72 kg, how much enoximone 2.5 mg/mL would he have been administered after 25 minutes?

  A   0.576 mL
  B   7.2 mL
  C   72 mL
  D   14.4 mL
  E   144 mL

5   Regarding the following extract from a prescription:

   Prednisolone 5 mg e/c tablets
   Take 45 mg on day 1 reducing the dose every other day by 5 mg until a dose of 5 mg is reached for 3 days

   How many prednisolone 5mg e/c tablets will you dispense?

  A   45
  B   47
  C   59
  D   73
  E   91

6   121 mg of quinine sulphate is equivalent to 100 mg of quinine anhydrous base. Estimate the molecular weight of quinine dihydrochloride given that the molecular weight of quinine anhydrous base is 324 g/mol.

  A   122 g/mol
  B   162 g/mol
  C   324 g/mol
  D   395 g/mol
  E   412 g/mol

7   Calculate the weight of salbutamol sulphate which contains 4 mg of salbutamol base:

   **Molecular weights**
   Salbutamol: $C_{13}H_{21}NO_3 = 239$ × 2
   Salbutamol sulphate: $(C_{13}H_{21}NO_3)_2H_2SO_4 = 577$ ✓ 4

  A   2.00 mg
  B   4.42 mg
  C   4.83 mg
  D   8.00 mg
  E   9.66 mg

8   What volume of 96% v/v alcohol is required to produce 8 L of 70% v/v alcohol?

    A   5833 mL
    B   6222 mL
    C   7000 mL
    D   7200 mL
    E   10 971 mL

9   Mr Q gives you a prescription for 450 g of 0.1% w/w dithranol in Lassar's paste. Calculate the weight of dithranol needed for this prescription.

    A   0.045 mg
    B   0.45 mg
    C   4.5 mg
    D   45 mg
    E   450 mg

10  Mr J, a 47-year-old man who weighs 75 kg, has been admitted to hospital for a short surgical procedure. The surgeon decides to give Mr J an intramuscular injection of ketamine 6.5 mg/kg. Calculate the minimum period of anaesthesia which Mr J will receive:

    A   6 minutes 48 seconds
    B   7 minutes 20 seconds
    C   7 minutes 48 seconds
    D   8 minutes 20 seconds
    E   8 minutes 48 seconds

11  What is the percentage strength of a 1.2 L solution containing 1 *Permitab* tablet?

    A   0.0033% w/v
    B   0.033% w/v
    C   0.33% w/v
    D   3.3% w/v
    E   33% w/v

12 Approximately how many millimoles of sodium ions are present in 250 mL of sodium chloride solution 0.64% w/v?

**Atomic weights**
Sodium = 23 g/mol
Chlorine = 35.5 g/mol

    A   0.0274 mmol
    B   0.16 mmol
    C   1.6 mmol
    D   2.74 mmol
    E   27.4 mmol

13 Given that 14 drops of *Dalivit* multivitamin mixture is equivalent to an 0.6 mL dose, how many vitamin A units are present in 21 drops of this mixture?

    A   2500 units
    B   3333 units
    C   5000 units
    D   7500 units
    E   10,000 units

14 Mrs K has been taking *Peptac* suspension, 10 mL t.d.s for 2 weeks. How many millimoles of sodium ions has she received?

    A   86.8 mmol
    B   130.2 mmol
    C   260.4 mmol
    D   520.8 mmol
    E   2604 mmol

15 How much potassium chloride is required to prepare 1250 mL of a solution containing 8 mmol of potassium ions in every 5 mL?

**Atomic weights**
Potassium = 39 g/mol
Chlorine = 35.5 g/mol

    A   0.149 g
    B   149 mg
    C   1490 mg
    D   149 g
    E   1490 g

16  *Tagamet* syrup contains the $H_2$-receptor antagonist cimetidine. How much cimetidine is required to prepare 3 L of the syrup?

    A   0.12 g
    B   1.2 g
    C   12 g
    D   1.2 kg
    E   0.12 kg

17  How much adrenaline is required to make 400 mL of a 1 in 1000 preparation?

    A   0.4 mg
    B   40 mg
    C   400 mg
    D   4 g
    E   40 g

18  It is 4.30 p.m. on your ward and a doctor asks you to calculate the volume of eptifibatide that a patient has received since 7.30 a.m. You know that the patient weighs 75 kg and that the infusion device is still set at delivering a 2 micrograms/kg/min dose. What volume of eptifibatide has the patient received so far?

    A   40.5 mL
    B   81 mL
    C   96 mL
    D   107 mL
    E   108 mL

19  Drug B has a half-life of 4 hours. If the initial plasma level of drug B is 400 mg/L, what is the plasma level of this drug after 16 hours?

    A   12.5 mg/L
    B   12.75 mg/L
    C   18.5 mg/L
    D   18.75 mg/L
    E   25 mg/L

20 Which one of the following regimens provides 110 mg of elemental iron daily?

    A   *Galfer* syrup 7.5 mL b.d.
    B   ferrous gluconate 300 mg tablets t.d.s.   –
    C   *Sytron* elixir 10 mL b.d.
    D   *Pregaday* tablet o.d.
    E   *Ferrograd* Folic tablet o.d. –

21 Regarding the following extract from a prescription:

    Amiodarone 200 mg tablets
    Take 200 mg t.d.s. for 1 week then
    take 200 mg b.d. for 1 week then
    take 200 mg o.d. for 1 week

How many amiodarone 200 mg tablets will you supply?

    A   28
    B   42
    C   56
    D   98
    E   101

22 A 6-year-old boy who weighs 19 kg is admitted to hospital after taking an overdose of paracetamol tablets. The ward doctor decides to start him on an intravenous infusion of acetylcysteine. Calculate the mass of acetylcysteine which is present in the initial dose for this patient:

    A   0.6 g
    B   1.14 g
    C   1.2 g
    D   11.4 g
    E   12 g

23 Calculate the total volume of *Immukin* subcutaneous injection needed for a patient with a body surface area of 1.6 m$^2$ for 7 days' treatment:

    A   0.1 mL
    B   0.4 mL
    C   0.8 mL
    D   1.2 mL
    E   4 mL

**24** A 28-year-old man who weighs 64 kg has taken an overdose of drug X. Given that the current serum level of drug X is 18 mg/L and that it has a clearance of 0.025 L/kg/h, calculate the amount of drug which will be removed from his body after 12 hours:

    A   3.46 mg
    B   34.56 mg
    C   345.6 mg
    D   3.456 g
    E   30.46 g

**25** *Duraphat* weekly dental rinse contains 0.2% sodium fluoride. How many milligrams of fluoride ions are present in a single weekly dose? Given:

Sodium fluoride 2.2 mg = fluoride ion 1 mg

    A   2 mg
    B   9.09 mg
    C   20 mg
    D   90.9 mg
    E   200 mg

**26** Mrs J is a patient on your ward who has recently developed a bacterial infection. Her doctor wishes to start her on cefalexin and asks you for advice on a suitable dose. After checking Mrs J's medical notes you find out that her serum creatinine is 100 micromol/L, that she weighs 54 kg and that she is 74 years old.

$$\text{Estimated creatinine clearance(mL/min)} = \frac{1.04 \times (140 - \text{age}) \times \text{weight(kg)}}{\text{Serum creatinine (micromol/L)}}$$

Which one of the following is the maximum daily dose that could be given to Mrs J?

    A   0.75 g
    B   1 g
    C   1.5 g
    D   2.75 g
    E   3 g

27  500 mL of benzalkonium chloride 5% w/v is required. You only have benzalkonium chloride 50% w/v in stock. What volume of this stock solution is required to prepare the 5% w/v solution?

    A    5 mL
    B    10 mL
    C    50 mL
    D    60 mL
    E    80 mL

28  You receive the following prescription:

    Fusidic acid ointment 0.2% w/w
    Use as directed
    Supply 60 g

Given that fusidic acid is available as a 2% w/w ointment, calculate the mass of fusidic acid 2% w/w which is required to produce 60 g of 0.2% w/w ointment:

    A    0.6 g
    B    1.2 g
    C    6 g
    D    12 g
    E    20 g

29  Mrs Y is a 52-year-old woman who weighs 75 kg. She has been admitted to hospital for cardiac surgery. She is prescribed dobutamine hydrochloride 2.5 micrograms/kg/min intravenous infusion. Calculate the rate of infusion for this preparation, given that dobutamine hydrochloride is administered as a 5 mg/mL solution.

    A    0.0375 mL/h
    B    2.25 mL/h
    C    22.5 mL/h
    D    50 mL/h
    E    225 mL/h

30 Regarding the following extract from a prescription:

> Dicycloverine hydrochloride 10 mg/5 mL syrup
> 15 mg t.d.s. for 8 days

Calculate the total volume of the dicycloverine hydrochloride 10 mg/ 5 mL syrup to dispense:

    A    18 mL
    B    20 mL
    C    50 mL
    D    90 mL
    E    180 mL

31 Given that the molecular weight of potassium chloride is 74.5 g/mol, calculate the mass of potassium chloride which is required to prepare 3 L of a solution containing 1 mmol/mL:

    A    0.2235 g
    B    0.447 g
    C    22.35 g
    D    44.7 g
    E    223.5 g

32 An intravenous infusion, containing 0.5 g in 250 mL of drug X, is prepared to be administered to a patient on your ward at 8 a.m. Calculate the flow rate, in drops per minute, required to infuse 25 mg of drug X per minute (the infusion device is set at 20 drops/mL):

    A    20
    B    25
    C    50
    D    125
    E    250

33 Calculate the mass of sodium chloride which is present in 250 mL sodium chloride 0.5% w/v infusion:

    A    0.5 g
    B    1 g
    C    1.25 g
    D    1.5 g
    E    2 g

*The answers for this section are on pp. 185–189.*

## MULTIPLE COMPLETION QUESTIONS

Each one of the questions or incomplete statements in this section is followed by three responses. For each question, ONE or MORE of the responses is/are correct. Decide which of the responses is/are correct, then choose:

A  if 1, 2 and 3 are correct
B  if 1 and 2 only are correct
C  if 2 and 3 only are correct
D  if 1 only is correct
E  if 3 only is correct

| Summary | | | | |
|---------|---------|-----------|--------|--------|
| A | B | C | D | E |
| 1, 2, 3 | 1, 2 only | 2, 3 only | 1 only | 3 only |

1  You are asked to prepare the following formulation:

| | |
|---|---|
| **Morphine hydrochloride** | 10 mg |
| **Nitrazepam** | 2.5 mg |
| **Alcohol (95%)** | 0.9 mL |
| **Rose water single strength** | 1.5 mL |
| **Water** | up to 5 mL |
| **Supply** | 250 mL |

You have the following ingredients in stock:
Morphine hydrochloride 10 mg
Nitrazepam 5 mg
Alcohol (90%)
Rose water double strength

Which of the following quantities of the available ingredients is/are correct for preparing the required formula?

1    25 nitrazepam 5 mg tablets
2    42.6 mL alcohol (90%)
3    150 mL of rose water double strength

2    Which of the following regimens would provide a patient with 310 mg of chloroquine base weekly?

1    *Nivaquine* syrup 20 mL
2    *Malarivon* syrup 31 mL
3    *Avloclor* × 2 tablets

3    A family of two adults and an 8-year-old child (who weighs 26 kg) ask for your advice on malaria prevention as they are going on a 3-week holiday to Mexico next week. After a thorough discussion with the family you find out that they are all suitable for treatment with *Avloclor* tablets. Which of the following statements is/are true?

1    the total number of tablets which you will supply is 54
2    the total amount of chloroquine base which the family will receive is 6.82 g
3    the child will receive approximately 71.5 mg/kg of chloroquine base over the full course of treatment

4    Mrs J is a 37-year-old woman with an anal fissure. She is prescribed *Rectogesic* 0.4% rectal ointment and is told to apply 2.5 cm of the ointment to the anal canal every 12 hours until the pain subsides. Which of the following statements is/are correct?

1    Mrs J is removing 37.5 mg of the ointment with each application
2    42 mg of glyceryl trinitrate would be applied, if *Rectogesic* were used continuously for 2 weeks
3    *Rectogesic* should be discarded 8 weeks after first opening

5    You are asked to prepare 9 × 5 mg of drug X powders diluted with lactose. You ascertain the final weight of each powder to be 120 mg and decide to calculate for one powder in excess. Which of the following total quantity/quantities would you use?

1    45 mg of drug X and 1035 mg of lactose
2    50 mg of drug X and 1500 mg of lactose
3    50 mg of drug X and 1150 mg of lactose

6 Which of the following is/are true with regard to parenteral preparations which are used to treat electrolyte disturbances?

   1 Glucose infusions can be used initially in patients with severe hypokalaemia

   2 Potassium chloride 15% concentrate contains 1 mol of $K^+$ ions in 0.5 L of infusion

   3 2 mL of potassium chloride concentrate 15% is required to be added to 500 mL of sodium chloride 0.9% infusion to produce a concentration of 8 mmol potassium ions per litre

7 Which of the following statements is/are true regarding the use of papaveretum injection for a 3-month-old child who weighs 6 kg?

   1 0.06 mL of papaveretum 15.4 mg/mL injection should be administered to this child

   2 The child's dose is equivalent to 600 micrograms of anhydrous morphine per millilitre

   3 Papaveretum non-parenteral preparation diluted to 1 ppm is a CD POM

8 Which of the following statements is/are true?

   1 A person weighing 58 kg with an eGFR of 8 mL/min/1.73 $m^2$ may be given zidovudine 232 mg in 4 divided doses

   2 A patient with severe renal impairment who has been prescribed perindopril erbumine for 2 weeks will receive a total supply of $7 \times 2$ mg tablets

   3 The maximum daily dose of amisulpride for the treatment of an acute psychotic episode in a patient with severe renal impairment is 0.6 g

9 Mr P is a 54-year-old man who weighs 67.5 kg. He is prescribed drug X 4 mg/kg/day to be administered by intravenous infusion in divided doses every 8 hours. Which of the following doses are suitable for Mr P?

   1 90 mL of a 1 mg/mL infusion every 8 hours

   2 30 mL of a 3 mg/mL infusion every 8 hours

   3 270 mL of a 3 mg/mL infusion every 8 hours

10 Regarding *Dermol* cream, which of the following statements is/are true?

   1 45 g contains 45 mg of benzalkonium chloride

   2 90 g contains 9 g of isopropyl myristate

   3 125 g contains 0.125 g of chlorhexidine hydrochloride

11  When the fluoride content in drinking water falls below the limit spec-
    ified in the BNF, fluoride supplements may be taken. Which of the
    following fluoride content(s) is/are lower than the BNF recommended
    limits?

    1   0.03 g of sodium fluoride in 50 L water
    2   35 L of sodium fluoride 0.001% w/v solution which is diluted with
        35 L of water
    3   10 L of sodium fluoride 1 in 200 000 solution which is diluted with
        40 L of water

*The answers for this section are on pp. 190–192.*

## CLASSIFICATION QUESTIONS

In this section, for each numbered question, select the one lettered option that most closely corresponds to the answer. Within each group of questions each lettered option may be used once, more than once or not at all.

Questions 1–3 concern the volume of morphine salts to be administered by subcutaneous or intramuscular injection:

A   0.04 mL
B   0.14 mL
C   0.24 mL
D   0.25 mL
E   1.4 mL

Which of the above is the appropriate initial injection volume to be given to the following patients?

1   20 mg/mL of morphine sulphate for a 3-year-old child who weighs 14 kg to treat acute pain
2   15 mg/mL of morphine sulphate for an 8-year-old child who weighs 25 kg as premedication
3   10 mg/mL of morphine sulphate to a 25-day-old baby who weighs 4 kg to treat acute pain

Questions 4 and 5 concern the following quantities:

A   0.0025 g
B   0.025 g
C   0.25 g
D   2.5 g
E   25 g

Which of the above is the weight of:

4   adrenaline present in 25 mL of a 1 in 1000 injection?
5   sodium bicarbonate in 1.25 L of a 0.2% w/v solution?

Questions 6 and 7 concern the following quantities of sodium chloride:

    A   0.025 g
    B   2 g
    C   2.5 g
    D   5 g
    E   7.5 g

Which of the above quantities would be required to make:

6   500 mL of a 1 in 200 solution
7   40 mL of a solution which when diluted with 110 mL of water results in a 5% w/v solution

*The answers for this section are on p. 193.*

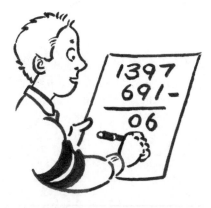

# Calculation answers

## SIMPLE COMPLETION ANSWERS

**1 A**

Concentrated chloroform water is 40 times single strength, hence $200 \div 40 = 5$ mL concentrated chloroform water is needed.

**2 D**

$(250 \times 0.65) \div 0.8 = 203.125$ micrograms daily of digoxin elixir. See BNF, Chapter 2 (Cardiovascular system), section 2.1.1. Cardiac glycosides. Elixir contains 50 micrograms/mL digoxin, hence 203.125/50 = 4.06 mL ~ 4 mL.

**3 E**

0.05 g in 100 g, 0.005 g in 10 g, 0.02 g in 40 g = 20 mg in 40 g.

**4 D**

The dose for Mr A is $72 \times 20 = 1440$ micrograms/min. 1 mL of the infusion contains 2.5 mg enoximone, hence the infusion rate for Mr A is $(1440 \div 2500) \times 1000 = 0.576$ mL in 1 minute = 14.4 mL in 25 minutes.

**√5 E**

Dosing regimen from day 1 is as follows: 45 mg, 45 mg, 40 mg, 40 mg, 35 mg, 35 mg, 30 mg, 30 mg, 25 mg, 25 mg, 20 mg, 20 mg, 15 mg, 15 mg, 10 mg, 10 mg, 5 mg, 5 mg and 5 mg. The total is 91 prednisolone 5 mg e/c tablets.

**⊤6 D**

100 mg quinine anhydrous base is equivalent to 122 mg quinine dihydrochloride. The molecular weight of quinine dihydrochloride is $(122/100) \times 324 = 395.28$ g/mol ~ 395 g/mol. See BNF, Chapter 5 (Infections), section 5.4.1, Antimalarials, Quinine.

**7 C**

Based on the molecular formulae, we can see that salbutamol sulphate contains 2 mol salbutamol base. Thus the answer can be calculated as $(4\,mg \times 577) \div (2 \times 239) = 4.83\,mg$ salbutamol sulphate.

**8 A**

$(8 \times 70\%) \div 96\% = 5.833\,L = 5833\,mL.$

**9 E**

$0.1\,g$ dithranol in $100\,g$ Lassar's paste. Thus: $(450 \times 0.1) \div 100 = 0.45\,g = 450\,mg$ dithranol is present in $450\,g$ Lassar's paste.

**10 C**

Ketamine $10\,mg/kg$ usually produces a minimum of 12 minutes of surgical anaesthesia. Hence $6.5\,mg/kg$ will produce a minimum of $(6.5 \div 10) \times 12 = 7.8$ minutes $= 7$ minutes and 48 seconds. See BNF, Chapter 15 (Anaesthesia), section 15.1.1, Intravenous anaesthetics, Ketamine.

**11 B**

See BNF, Chapter 13 (Skin), section 13.11.6, Oxidisers and dyes. Permitabs solution tablet contains $400\,mg$ potassium permanganate. $(400\,mg \div 1000) \div (1.2\,L \times 1000) = 0.033\,\%w/v.$

**12 E**

$(0.64 \div 100) \times 250 = 1.6\,g$ sodium chloride. $1.6 \div 58.5 = 0.0274\,mol = 27.4$ millimol sodium ions ($1:1$ ratio, hence equal to sodium chloride).

**13 D**

*Dalivit* multivitamin drops contain 5000 units vitamin A in every $0.6\,mL$ dose. This is equivalent to 14 drops of *Dalivit*, hence 21 drops contain $5000 + 2500 = 7500$ units vitamin A. See BNF, Chapter 9 (Nutrition and blood), section 9.6.7, Multivitamin preparations, *Dalivit*.

**14 C**

*Peptac* contains $3.1\,mmol\ Na^+$ in every $5mL$. Total amount of sodium ions taken by Mrs K is: $3.1 \times 2 \times 3 \times 14 = 260.4\,mmol$. See BNF, Chapter 1 (Gastro-intestinal system), section 1.1.2, Compound alginates and proprietary indigestion preparations, Alginate raft-forming oral suspensions, *Peptac*.

**15 D**

Number of moles of potassium chloride $= (8 \div 5) \times 1250 = 2000$ mmol $K^+ = KCl$ ($1:1$ ratio). Mass of $KCl = (35.5 + 39) \times 2000 = 149\,000\,mg = 149\,g$.

**16 E**

*Tagamet* syrup contains cimetidine $200\,mg/5\,mL$, hence the mass of cimetidine that is required to prepare $3\,L$ of the syrup is: $(200 \div 5) \times 3000 = 120\,000\,mg = 120\,g = 0.12\,kg$. See BNF, Chapter 1 (Gastrointestinal system), section 1.3.1, $H_2$-receptor antagonists, Cimetidine.

**17 C**

$1\,g$ adrenaline is present in $1000\,mL$ of preparation, hence $(1 \div 1000) \times 400 = 0.4\,g = 400\,mg$.

**18 E**

Dose for the patient is $75 \times 2 = 150$ micrograms/min. $150 \times 60 \times 9 = 81\,000$ micrograms in 9 hours. The infusion contains $750$ micrograms eptifibatide in $1\,mL$, hence the volume administered over 9 hours is $81000 \div 750 = 108\,mL$. See BNF, Chapter 2 (Cardiovascular system), section 2.9, Antiplatelet drugs, Eptifibatide.

**19 E**

$16 \div 4 = 4$ half-lives, after which the plasma concentration of drug B is $25\,mg/L$.

**20 C**

*Sytron* elixir contains $27.5\,mg$ elemental iron in each $5\,mL$. Hence, $27.5 \times 2 \times 2 = 110\,mg$. See BNF, Chapter 9 (Nutrition and blood), section 9.1.1.1, Oral iron.

**21 B**

$(1 \times 3 \times 7) + (1 \times 2 \times 7) + (1 \times 1 \times 7) = 42$ of amiodarone $200\,mg$ tablets.

**22 D**

The initial dose of acetylcysteine for a child whose weight is less than $20\,kg$ is $3\,mL/kg$ over 15 minutes. Hence the volume of a $200\,mg/mL$ infusion to be given to this boy is $19 \times 3 = 57\,mL$. The mass of acetylcysteine in this volume is $57 \times 200 = 11\,400\,mg = 11.4\,g$. See BNF, Emergency treatment of poisoning, Specific drugs, Analgesics (non-opioid), Acetylcysteine.

23 D

*Immukin* dose is 50 micrograms/m$^2$ three times a week. Total weekly dose for this patient is $50 \times 1.6 \times 3 = 240$ micrograms. The volume of *Immukin* injection 200 micrograms/mL required is $240 \div 200 = 1.2$ mL. See BNF, Chapter 8 (Malignant disease and immunosuppression), section 8.2.4, Other immunomodulating drugs, Interferon gamma-1b.

24 C

$0.025 \times 64 = 1.6$ L/hour.    $1.6 \times 18 = 28.8$ mg/hour.    $28.8 \times 12 = 345.6$ mg.

25 B

Mass of sodium fluoride in a 10 mL weekly rinse $= (0.2 \div 100) \times 10 = 0.02$ g $= 20$ mg. $20 \div 2.2 = 9.09$ mg fluoride ions in each 10 mL rinse. See BNF, Chapter 9 (Nutrition and blood), section 9.5.3, Fluoride, Fluorides, Mouthwashes, *Duraphat*.

26 C

Substituting into the formula $= (1.04 \times 66 \times 54) \div 100 = 37.1$ mL/min/1.73 m$^2$. The BNF states (see BNF, Chapter 5 (Infections), section 5.1.2.1, Cephalosporins, Cefalexin, Renal impairment) that if eGFR is 10–40 mL/min/1.73 m$^2$, the maximum daily dose is 1.5 g.

27 C

$(0.05 \times 500) \div 0.5 = 50$ mL benzalkonium chloride 50% w/v.

28 C

$(0.002 \times 60) \div 0.02 = 6$ g.

29 B

$2.5 \times 75 = 187.5$ micrograms/min $= 0.1875$ mg/min.
$0.1875 \times 60 = 11.25$ mg/hour.
$11.25 \div 5 = 2.25$ mL/hour.

30 E

10 mg in 5 mL, thus 15 mg in 7.5 mL.
For the total course of treatment, supply: $7.5 \times 3 \times 8 = 180$ mL.

**31 E**

$1 \times 3 \times 1000 = 3000$ mmol.

$(3000/1000) \times 74.5 = 223.5$ g.

**32 E**

$(25 \times 250) \div 500 = 12.5$ mL/min. $12.5 \times 20 = 250$ drops per minute.

**33 C**

$(250 \times 0.5) \div 100 = 1.25$ g sodium chloride.

## MULTIPLE COMPLETION ANSWERS

### 1 D

250 mL supply is 50 times the 5 mL formulation.

1  Total mass of nitrazepam: $2.5 \times 50 = 125$ mg in 250 mL
   $5 \times 25 = 125$ mg nitrazepam 5 mg tablets, hence correct.

2  Total volume of alcohol (95%): $0.9 \times 50 = 45$ mL in 250 mL
   $(95\% \times 45) \div 90\% = 47.5$ mL alcohol 90%, hence 42.6 mL
   incorrect.

3  Total volume of rose water single-strength: $1.5 \times 50 = 75$ mL
   Double-strength rose water is twice single-strength, hence correct answer is $75$ mL $\div 2 = 37.5$ mL double-strength rose water, not 150 mL: incorrect.

### 2 C

*Nivaquine* syrup: $(50$ mg $\div 5) \times 20 = 200$ mg; *Malarivon* syrup: $(50$ mg $\div 5) \times 31 = 310$ mg; *Avloclor* $\times 2$ tablets $= 155 \times 2 = 310$ mg. See BNF, Chapter 5 (Infections), section 5.4.1, Antimalarials, Chloroquine.

### 3 C

Prophylactic regimen: once weekly 1 week before, during and for 4 weeks after return
Adult dose: 155 mg (chloroquine base) $\times 2$ *Avloclor* tablets
Child dose: (8–13 years and weighing 25–45 kg) 232.5 mg chloroquine base $\times 1.5$ *Avloclor* tablet

1  Total number of *Avloclor* tablets: both adults: $2 \times 8 \times 2 = 32$ tablets + child who weighs 26 kg (8–13 years body weight 25–45 kg, 232.5 mg once weekly if tablets used. This equates to $232.5 \div 155 = 1.5$ tablets). Hence total number of tablets for the family is $32 + (1.5 \times 8) = 44$ tablets, therefore statement 1 is incorrect.

2  Total chloroquine base which you will supply $= 155 \times 44 = 6820$ mg $= 6.82$ g: correct.

3  Child will receive 232.5 mg (chloroquine base) $\times 8$ weeks $= 1860$ mg. $1860 \div 26$ kg $\sim 71.5$ mg/kg: correct.

See BNF, Chapter 5 (Infections), section 5.4.1, Antimalarials, Chloroquine.

**4  A**

 1   0.4 g GTN in 100 g ointment, 1.5 mg of GTN per 2.5 cm application. Amount of ointment removed with each application: $1.5 \div 4 = 0.375$ g $= 375$ mg: correct.
 2   1.5 mg $\times 2$ applications per day $\times 14$ days $= 42$ mg GTN: correct.
 3   Correct. See BNF, Chapter 1 (Gastro-intestinal system), section 1.7.4, Management of anal fissures, Glyceryl trinitrate.

**5  E**
Total powders $= 10$. Total amount of drug $X = 5 \times 10 = 50$ mg. Total amount of lactose $= (120 - 5) \times 10 = 1150$ mg.

**6  C**
Statement 1 is incorrect because the use of glucose infusions at the start of potassium replacement therapy may cause a further decrease in the plasma potassium concentration.
Statement 2 is correct: potassium chloride 15% concentrate contains 2 mmol/mL $K^+$ ions, hence, in a 0.5 L infusion: $2 \times 500 = 1000$ mmol $= 1$ mol $K^+$ ions.
Statement 3 is correct: $(0.008 \times 500 \text{ mL}) \div 2 \text{ mmol} = 2$ mL.
See BNF, Chapter 9 (Nutrition and blood), section 9.2.2.1, Electrolytes and water.

**7  B**
BNF dose 1–12 months 154 micrograms/kg, for this child: $154 \times 6 = 924$ micrograms.

 1   Injection $924 \div (15\,400) = 0.06$ mL.
 2   Papaveretum 15.4 mg/mL is equivalent to 10 mg anhydrous morphine/mL. Hence, $(924/15.4) \times 10 = 600$ micrograms anhydrous morphine per mL.
 3   Papaveretum non-parenteral preparation diluted to 1 ppm is a CD Inv. See MEP, section 1.3, Alphabetical list of medicines for human use.

See BNF, Chapter 4 (Central nervous system), section 4.7.2, Opioid analgesics, Papaveretum.

**8  B**

 1   BNF: 'zidovudine IV 1 mg/kg in 3–4 divided doses'. Patient: $58 \times 1 \times 4 = 232$ mg in 4 divided doses.

2 Severe renal impairment is classified as an eGFR of 15–29 mL/min/1.73 m². BNF dose is 2 mg once daily on alternate days if eGFR is 15–30 mL/min/1.73 m². Hence, 14-day supply = 7 × 2 mg tablets.

3 Use one-third of the dose of amisulpride if eGFR is 10–30 mL/min/1.73 m². BNF maximum daily dose of amisupride = 1.2 g, 1.2 g ÷ 3 ≠ 0.6 g.

See individual BNF entries, Renal impairment.

**9 B**

1 67.5 × 4 = 270 mg drug X daily for Mr P
270 mg ÷ 3 = 90 mg every 8 hours
90 mL of a 1 mg/mL infusion every 8 hours: correct.

2 90 ÷ 3 = 30 mL of 3 mg/mL infusion every 8 hours: correct.

3 Incorrect.

**10 A**

1 (45 × 0.1) ÷ 100 = 0.045 g = 45 mg benzalkonium chloride.

2 (90 × 10) ÷ 100 = 9 g isopropyl myristate.

3 (125 × 0.1) ÷ 100 = 0.125 g chlorhexidine hydrochloride.

See BNF, Chapter 13 (Skin), section 13.2.1, Emollients, With antimicrobials, *Dermol*.

**11 D**
See BNF, Chapter 9 (Nutrition and blood), section 9.5.3, Fluoride. Fluoride supplements may be taken if the fluoride content in drinking water falls below 700 micrograms/L (0.7 ppm).

1 Fluoride content = (0.03 ÷ 50 000) × 1 000 000 = 0.6 ppm, hence, lower than BNF limit.

2 Fluoride content: (0.001 ÷ 100) × 35 000 = 0.35 g. [0.35 ÷ (35 000 + 35 000)] × 1 000 000 = 5 ppm, hence, higher than BNF limit.

3 Fluoride content: (1 ÷ 200 000) × 10 000 = 0.05 g. [0.05 ÷ (10 000 + 40 000)] × 1 000 000 = 1 ppm, hence, higher than BNF limit.

## CLASSIFICATION QUESTION ANSWERS

**1  B**

See BNF, Chapter 4 (Central nervous system), section 4.7.2, Opioid analgesics, Morphine salts, Acute pain. $14 \times 200 = 2800$ micrograms for this patient. The corresponding volume of morphine sulphate injection is: $2800 \div 20000 = 0.14$ mL every 4 hours.

**2  D**

See BNF, Chapter 4 (Central nervous system), section 4.7.2, Opioid analgesics, Morphine salts, Premedication. $150 \times 25 = 3750$ micrograms for this patient. The corresponding volume of morphine sulphate injection is: $3750 \div 15000 = 0.25$ mL.

**3  A**

See BNF, Chapter 4 (Central nervous system), section 4.7.2, Opioid analgesics, Morphine salts, Acute pain. $4 \times 100 = 400$ micrograms for this patient. The corresponding volume of morphine sulphate injection is: $400 \div 10000 = 0.04$ mL every 6 hours.

**4  B**

$25 \div 1000 = 0.025$ g adrenaline in 25 mL.

**5  D**

$(1.25 \times 0.2) \div 100 = 2.5$ g sodium bicarbonate in 1.25 L.

**6  C**

$500 \div 200 = 2.5$ g sodium chloride.

**7  E**

$[(40 + 110) \times 5] \div 100 = 7.5$ g sodium chloride.

# Index

abciximab, 48
absence seizures, 32
Acarbose, 150
Accupro 20 mg tablets, 37
ACE *see* angiotensin-converting enzymes
acemetacin, 29
acetylcysteine, 174, 187
acetylsalicylic acid, 14, 47, 105, 121,
    125, 156, 161
aciclovir, 34
acitretin, 36, 72
Acnamino MR capsules, 35
acne, 83, 108, 127, 133
acrivastine 8 mg capsules, 128
active liver disease, 104, 146
Acumed patches, 34, 70
acute gout attacks, 47, 105, 147
acute leg pain, 77
acute lymphoblastic leukaemia, 31
acute porphyria, 13
acute psychotic episode, 181
Adcal D$_3$ effervescent tablets, 35
adrenal suppression, 123, 158
adrenaline, 173, 183, 187, 193
Advagraf, 57
advanced prostate cancer, 29
advanced services, 98, 144
advisory labels, 5, 19, 37, 71, 83, 124,
    129, 159
agranulocytosis, 131
alcohol
    acitretin, 72
    avoidance warnings, 37
    calculations, 179, 190
    cautionary and advisory labels, 37, 124
    denatured alcohols, 22, 39, 42, 43
    dependent patients, 31, 56
    etretinate, 72
    recommended limit, 106
    teratogenicity, 36
    volume of, 171
    withdrawal, 123, 158
alcometasone dipropionate, 169
aldosterone antagonists, 122, 157
alert cards, 103
alginate raft-forming oral suspensions,
    186
allergies, 14, 25, 35, 78, 124
Alli, 104, 146
Allopurinol, 47, 118, 147, 154
Amdipharm, 31
Amias tablets, 15
amikacin sulphate, IV, 3
amiloride, 32
aminoglycoside, 96
aminophylline, 124
amiodarone, 32, 120, 122, 124, 132,
    140, 155, 157, 174, 187
amisulpride, 181, 192
amitriptyline, 81, 102, 124
amoxicillin, 122, 134
amphetamines, 61
ampicillin therapy, 45
anabolic steroids, 53
anaemia, 126
anaesthesia, 87, 171, 186
anal fissures, 180
analgesics, 123, 193
anaphylactic reactions, 20, 156
Andrews Liver Salts, 42
angina, 83
angiotensin-converting enzymes (ACE),
    31, 126, 137, 165
Angitil SR 90 mg capsules, 37
anhydrous morphine, 191
anorexia, 132

Antepsin, 36
antiandrogens, 148
antiarrhythmic drugs, 124
antibiotic-induced colitis, 45, 83, 133, 165
antibiotics, 25, 84, 111, 121
anticoagulants, 30, 132, 139
antidepressants, 13, 28, 63, 126, 134, 136, 166
antidiabetic therapy, 112, 132
antidiarrhoea treatments, 97
antihistamines, 137
antimalarials, 21, 111
antimetics, 134
antimuscarinics, 83, 137, 139
antiplatelet drugs, 95, 125, 142, 156, 161
antipsychotics, 26, 118, 139, 154
aplastic anaemia, 126
Approved Classification and Labelling Guide, 42
arachis oil, 35, 71
Asasantin Retard, 26, 61
Asian ginseng, 97, 143
aspirin, 14, 47, 105, 121, 125, 156, 161
asthma attacks, 124
Astra Zeneca, 31
ataxia, 164
atenolol, 124, 134
atomic weights, 172
atorvastatin, 124, 140
atrial fibrillation, 83, 139
audits, 43, 116, 135, 166
authorised persons, 99, 112, 144
AV block, 31
Avloclor, 101, 180, 190
Avodart capsules, 37
Axorid, 30

Bach rescue cream, 42
bacteria, 6, 49, 114, 124, 133
bacterial infections, 175
bacteriostatic properties, 129
barbiturates, 14
Bard Biocath Hydrogel Coated Foley catheters, 50
barrier preparations, 30
beclometasone dipropionate, 128
benzalkonium chloride, 176, 188, 192
benzodiazepines, 123, 158

Benzphetamine, 55
beta-2 adrenoceptor antagonists, 134
beta-2 agonists, 124, 126, 142, 159
beta-blockers, 80, 81, 94, 119, 133, 138, 141
betamethasone inhalers, 102
bezoar formation, 72
bipolar disorder, 124, 126, 159
Bisoprolol, 78
bisphosphonates, 49
black dot interactions, 2, 4, 114, 152
blacklisted items, 30, 51, 146, 148
bleeding risks, 62, 105, 152
bleomycin, 56
blood, 12, 32, 97
blood–brain barrier, 130
blurred vision, 137, 139
body mass index (BMI), 61, 81, 104, 146
body surface area, 174
body temperature, 96
body weights, 61, 181
bone marrow suppression, 57, 60
borotannic complex, 33
bottle regulations, 21, 43, 58
bowel conditions, 50
breast-feeding, 4, 48
Bricanyl Turbohalers, 6, 49
brinzolamide, 29
broad-spectrum antibiotics, 43, 83, 133, 165
broken bulk claims, 10, 51
broken packages, 9, 51
broncospasm, 138
brotizolam, 34
Bug Buster Kit, 50
bumetanide, 122, 133, 157, 165
Buprenorphine, 153

Cabergoline, 71
cabinet storage, 39
calcitonin, 31
calcium, 32
calcium salts, 49
calculation questions, 169, 183
cannabinoids, 133
cannabis, 40
capsule colouration, 31
captopril, 32, 93
carbamazepine, 124, 148, 159
carbimazole, 24, 57, 60

Carbomer eye gel, 21
carcinogenicity, 52
Carmellose Gelatin Paste DPF, 61
catheters, 7, 50
cautionary and advisory labels, 5, 19, 37, 71, 83, 124, 129, 159
CE *see conformité européenne* mark
cefalexin, 175
cell membranes, 154
cerebral sensitivity, 32
cessation of medication, 12, 63, 136
CFC-free inhalers, 37
charges *see* prescription charges/fees
Chemicals (Hazard Information and Packaging for Supply) 2002, 23
chest infections, 86
child abuse, 117
child care agencies, 41
child-bearing potential, 36
childhood pyrexia, 96
chiropodists, 33
chlorhexidine hydrochloride, 192
chloroform, 40
chloroform water, 169, 185
Chloromycetin Redidrops, 36
chloroquine, 128, 180, 190
Cholestagel tablets, 36
cholestatic jaundice, 44
ciclosporin, 2, 36, 72, 142, 155
cimetidine, 52, 173, 187
ciprofloxacin, 86, 102, 123, 128, 157
Claritin, 78
classification questions, 29, 122, 183
clearance calculations, 175
clenbuterol, 33, 69
Clever Chek strips, 51
clindamycin, 133
clinical audits, 116, 135
clinical effectiveness, 162
clinical management plans, 112
clioquinol staining, 71, 145
clobetasone cream, 34
clomethiazole, 31
clonidine, 29, 164
*Clostridium difficile*, 49
clothes stains, 71, 145
clotting, blood, 97
clozapine, 32
co-amoxiclav, 124
co-careldopa, 125, 161

co-codamol, 124, 159
co-cyprindiol, 148
co-danthramer suspension, 124
co-fluampicil, 43
cocaine, 105
cod liver oil, 30
Codalax oral suspension, 37
code of ethics, 115, 117
codeine, 123, 124, 137, 158, 159
codeine phosphate, 164
Codipar caplets, 34, 70
coeliac disease, 128, 163
cold sores, 34
Colestyramine, 148
colistin, 29
colitis, 45, 83, 133, 165
colouration, 11, 30, 31, 37, 80, 102, 124, 137
combined oral contraceptives, 108, 110, 134, 149, 155
community pharmacies, 135
community practitioner nurses, 50, 121
community-acquired pneumonia, 25
compression hosiery, 122
concentrated chloroform water, 185
condoms, 26, 61
conducting clinical audits, 135
confidentiality, 17, 45, 55
*conformité européenne* (CE) mark, 100, 135, 145
constipation, 12, 30, 129, 134
contact lenses, 41
continuous improvement of quality and maintenance, 116
continuous intravenous infusion, 170
continuous professional development (CPD), 115
contraception
  acne treatment, 108
  amoxicillin, 134
  combined oral, 108, 110, 134, 149, 155
  condoms, 26, 61
  doxycycline, 155
  emergency supplies, 93, 99, 141
  FP10 form, 27
  isotretinoin, 60
  Marvelon, 120
  payment exemption, 27
  prescription charges, 138, 140
  Roaccutane capsules, 25

side-effects, 149
teratogenics, 60
contraindications, 1, 11, 21, 30, 31, 81
controlled drugs, 83, 93, 165
  cabinet storage, 39
  classification questions, 33, 123, 127
  clenbuterol, 33, 69
  Codipar caplets, 70
  community practitioner nurses, 156
  custody safety, 33, 43
  denaturing, 39
  destruction, 152
  dispensing instructions, 115
  electronic records, 40
  emergency supplies, 55, 123
  export licenses, 127
  Home Office advice, 39
  Home Secretary, 40
  import/export licenses, 127
  independent nurses, 156
  legal requirements, 40
  LSD, 70
  Nabilone, 133
  nurses, 156
  optometrists, 156
  OxyContin tablets, 39
  patient group direction, 43
  possession restrictions, 33
  prescription validity, 141
  record-keeping requirements, 94
  requisitions, 23
  restrictions on possession, 33
  temazepam, 132
  withdrawal of alcohol, 123
Convulex capsules, 35
convulsions, 123, 140, 157
cool place storage, 87
Cooley's anaemia, 126
corneal microdeposits, 122, 157
corticosteroids, 35
coughs, 94, 126
counterfeit medicines, 100
COX-1 enzyme inhibition, 125, 161
CPD *see* continuous professional development
Creon granules, 41
criminal convictions, 116, 153
custody safety, 33, 43
cyclizine, 125

Cyproterone acetate, 148
Cystofem sachets, 34
cytochrome P-450, 124, 125, 159, 160
cytotoxic-induced hyperuricaemia, 154

dacarbazine, 52
Daktarin oral gel, 34, 71
Dalivit multivitamins, 172, 186
Dalmane, 30, 36
danazol, 29
dangerous substance labelling, 42
dantrolene, 29
dasatinib, 31
daytime sleepiness, 12, 52
deep intramuscular injection, 139
deep-vein thrombosis, 130
Delph sun lotion SPF30, 51
denatured alcohol, 22, 39, 42, 43
dentists, 33, 61, 113
depot injections, 84, 118, 139, 154
depression, 13, 28, 63, 126, 134, 136, 166
dermatitis, 34
Dermol cream, 181
Dermovate, 35
destroying stock, 99, 144, 152
dexamfetamine poisoning, 26
diabetes, 96, 110, 112, 132, 142, 150, 155
diabetic ketoacidosis, 33
diagnostic tools, 28
diamorphine, 23, 33, 127
Dianette, 122, 148, 157
diarrhoea, 49, 97, 120, 143, 145
diazepam, 33, 41, 123, 127, 158, 162
diazoxide, 150
Diconal tablets, 35
dicycloverine hydrochloride syrup, 177
dietary supplements, 50
digoxin, 32, 78, 80, 122, 128, 157, 169, 185
  toxicity, 83, 104, 133, 138, 139, 145, 146, 165
dipyridamole, 32
direct contact avoidance, 103
disclosure of confidential information, 17, 55
discolouration, 30, 80, 102, 124, 137
discount not given (DNG), 27, 62, 108

discounts/discounting, 27, 62, 108, 148
dispensing prescriptions, 32, 35, 115
disulfiram, 56
dithranol, 171, 186
diuretics, 130, 138, 165
DNG *see* discount not given
dobutamine hydrochloride, 176
doctor–patient consultations, 25
doctor's emergency requests, 112
dopamine, 125, 132, 161
doripenem, 45
Dostinex tablets, 35
Dovonex cream, 37
doxorubicin, 56
doxycycline, 62, 83, 139, 146, 155
drinking water, 182, 192
driving or operating machinery, 106,
    124, 147
drop per minute flow rates, 177
drowsiness, 124
drug abuse, 98, 100, 105
drug combinations, 32
dry coughs, 94, 126
dry mouths, 58, 139
Duofilm paint, 37
Duraphat, 93, 175, 188
dust allergies, 78
duties of responsible pharmacists,
    21, 24, 45

E numbers, 36, 52, 72
echinacea, 126
eclampsia, 33
eGFR *see* estimated glomerular
    filtration rates
eggs, 20
electrolyte problems, 80, 143, 180
electronic records, 40
elemental iron, 174, 187
emergency supply, 16, 22, 26, 55, 59, 93,
    98, 99, 112, 117, 123, 141, 153, 158
enalapril, 78, 133, 137, 165
encephalopathy, 126, 129
endocarditis, 111
endometriosis, 7, 50
energy fat supplements, 3
enoxaparin, 32
enoximone, 170, 185
enzyme inducers, 155
enzyme inhibition, 161

epilepsy, 133, 158, 163
eptifibatide, 173
erdosteine, 32
erythromycin, 125, 155, 160
esmolol, 80
estimated glomerular filtration rates
    (eGFR), 32, 181, 192
Ethambutol, 85
ethosuximide, 31
etretinate, 72
Etrivex shampoo, 13
*Eumovate*, 35
exemption from fees, 27, 107, 148
expenses claims, 27, 62
export licenses, 34, 127, 136
extrapyramidal symptoms, 14,
    53, 154
eye drops, 36

facsimile transmissions, 113
Fasigyn tablets, 37
fat supplements, 3
fatal myocarditis, 32
fatal toxic syndrome, 20
faulty medical device reporting, 100
fees, 9, 27
    *see also* prescription charges/fees
fetal hypoxia, 31
fetal neural tube defects, 84
fever/feverfew, 126
finasteride, 57, 128
fine tremor, 95, 142
flammability cautions, 37
flow rates, 177
Flucloxacillin, 44, 139
Fludrocortisone, 149
fluoride, 32, 93, 175, 182, 188, 192
flutamide, 29
fluted bottles, 21, 43, 58
folic acid, 84, 139
food, 11, 95, 121, 124
forged prescriptions, 115, 152
Fosavance tablets, 36
fosinopril sodium, 36
FP10D forms, 8, 27, 115, 153
fraud, 115, 152
fridge temperature ranges, 87
fungal infections, 147
furosemide, 78, 131
fusidic acid, 176

G6PD *see* glucose-6-phosphate dehydrogenase
gabapentin, 24, 150
gastrointestinal upset, 142
gemfibrozil, 5
general sales list (GSL) items, 70, 113, 151
generic supply, 8, 135
gentamicin, 96, 142
gestation times, 96, 142
gingko, 126
ginseng, 97, 143
glandular fever, 45
glaucoma, 123
glomerular filtration rates, 13, 32, 181, 192
glucagon, 150
glucocorticoids, 110, 149, 158
glucosamine, 32
glucose infusions, 191
glucose-6-phosphate dehydrogenase (G6PD) deficiency, 19, 56, 129, 164
glycaemic control, 111, 150
glycerol, 164
glycerol suppositories, 129
glyceryl trinitrate (GTN), 24, 83, 138, 191
glycosylated haemoglobin, 125, 150
gout, 47, 105, 147, 154
GP14 (Scotland) prescription, 27
Gram-negative bacteria, 49
Gram-positive bacteria, 6, 49, 133
grapefruit juice, 36, 72, 140
green tea, 126
Grisol AF, 35
GSL *see* general sales list items
GTN *see* glyceryl trinitrate
Gygel, 36, 72
gynaecomastia, 122, 157

haemolysis, 11, 19, 56, 164
Haleraid, 30
half-lives, 173, 187
halitosis, 114
Hazardous Waste Regulations 2005, 99
headaches, 44, 139
heart failure, 80
heart rate, 134
*Helicobacter pylori* eradication, 124
hepatic encephalopathy, 126, 129

hepatic enzyme inducers, 155
hepatic impairment, 1, 4, 29, 32, 44, 47, 48
hepatitis, 5
hepatoxicity, 101, 145
herbal remedies, 126, 136
herpes zoster, 30
hexachlorophane, 15
hexobarbitone, 33
high sodium content, 6
high-energy fat supplements, 3
hirsutism, 148
Home Office, 34, 39, 136, 167
Home Secretary, 40
homeopathic products, 136
hormone replacement therapy (HRT), 7, 30
hosiery, 122, 138, 157
hospital-acquired pneumonia, 45
HRT *see* hormone replacement therapy
Humulin M3 pens, 145
hydrocortisone, 62
hyperglycaemia, 49
hyperkalaemia, 32
hypertension, 61, 81, 164
hyperthyroidism, 24
hyperuricaemia, 154
hypnotics, 30, 52
hypocalcaemia, 33
hypoglycaemia, 6, 8, 125, 150
hypokalaemia, 94, 122, 138, 142, 157, 165
hyponatraemia, 134
hypotension, 133, 137, 165
hypothyroidism, 110, 149
hysterectomy, 7, 50

ibuprofen, 124, 132
IDA *see* industrial denatured alcohol
illicit drug user supply, 100
Immukin subcutaneous injection, 174, 188
impetigo, 114, 127
import/export licenses, 34, 127, 136
indapamide, 11
independent nurses, 121, 156
Inderal-LA, 31
indigestion preparations, 35
Indivina, 30
industrial denatured alcohol (IDA), 22

industrial waste, 144
infertility, 29
inflammation, 30
influenza prevention, 10
infusion rates, 185
inhalers, 37, 124
installment supply, 153
insulin, 109, 125, 149, 161
intact uterus, 30
integrilin, 2
Interferon gamma-1b, 44
Internet, 46, 76
intestinal obstruction, 129
intramuscular injections, 61, 84, 139, 183
intraocular pressure, 29
intrauterine progesterone-only system, 48
intravenous infusions, 170, 177, 181
Intrinsa, 48
iodine, 25, 60
iron, 14, 32, 35, 126, 174, 187
irretrievable before disposal, 16
irritant effects, 129
ischaemic stroke, 26
isoniazid, 85, 119
isopropyl myristate, 192
isotretinoin, 60
itchy skin conditions, 102, 105

Joint Formulary Committee, 29

kaolin and morphine mixture, 127, 163
ketamine, 87, 171, 186
ketoacidosis, 33
Ketoconazole, 146

labelling, 15, 16, 23, 42, 93, 141
    cautionary and advisory, 5, 19, 37, 71, 83, 124, 129, 159
lactose, 180, 191
lactulose, 126, 128
Lanoxin injections, 24, 59
lansoprazole, 92, 141
Lassar's paste, 171, 186
laxatives, 129
leflunomide, 2
leg pain, 77
legal requirements, 16, 23, 40
legal validity, 87

legislation, 100
Lescol, 31
leukaemia, 31
levothyroxine, 32, 149
licenses, 7, 21, 34, 100, 107, 127, 136
lidocaine, 31
life-saving drugs, 15
lipophilic drugs, 118, 154
Lipostat, 13
lisinopril, 122
lithium, 77, 119, 124, 126, 128, 131, 154, 159, 161, 162, 164
liver disease, 104, 146, 147
liver failure, 121
local authority reports, 25
localised collection blood, 97
Locorten-Vioform, 35
long-term glycaemic control, 111
loop diuretics, 157
loratadine, 78
losartan, 126, 142
Losec MUPS tablets, 36
Lotemax, 36
low sodium content, 12, 50
low-molecular-weight heparins, 32
lower urinary tract infections, 121
lymphoblastic leukaemia, 31
lysergic acid diethylamide (LSD), 34, 70

macrolides, 125, 160
maculopapular rash, 45
magnesium, 32
magnesium phosphide, 42
maintenance standards, 116
malaria, 101, 111, 150, 180, 190
Malarivon syrup, 96, 190
malathion, 21, 110, 149
Mandanol 32 tablets, 34
mania, 126
manufacture, possession or supply, 34
Marevan, 30
Marvelon, 120, 155
master of ship, 42
Medicines Act 1968, 23
Medicines and Healthcare products
    Regulatory Agency (MHRA), 5, 25, 30, 52, 60, 136
Medicines Order 1979, 40
Medicines Regulations 1978, 43
Medicines Use Reviews (MUR), 144

mental diseases, 45
metformin, 123, 132, 142, 158
methadone, 98, 124, 143
methotrexate, 102, 126, 128, 131, 156
methylphenidate, 43
methylprednisolone, 33
methysergide, 47, 48
metopon, 34
metronidazole, 118, 124, 150
MHRA *see* Medicines and Healthcare
    products Regulatory Agency
Miacalcic, 31
Microgynon, 93, 135
Micronor, 140
Midazolam, 43
midwifes, 39
migraine, 29, 84, 102, 145
millimoles, 172
mineralocorticoid effects, 149
minerals, 32, 33
Minocyline tablets/capsules, 71
minor wounds, 30
Minoxidil solution, 148
mint-flavoured preparations, 37
Misoprostol, 145
Misuse of Drugs Act 1971, 40
Misuse of Drugs Regulations 2001, 127,
    162
modified-release form, 32, 140
Modrasone cream, 169
molecular weights, 86, 170, 185
moles, 187
monitoring
    diabetes, 150
    glycosylated haemoglobin, 125
    MHRA, 30, 48
    prothrombin time, 30
    SARSS, 22
Morhulin, 30
morphine, 112, 123, 124, 134, 158, 159
morphine hydrochloride, 179
morphine salts, 183, 193
morphine sulphate injection, 193
mouth preparations, 93, 175, 188
Moviprep oral powders, 35
MUR *see* Medicines Use Reviews
muscle pain, 124
Mycobutin, 30
mycordial infarction, 124
Myfortic tablets, 37

myocarditis, 32

nabilone, 23, 83, 127, 133, 165
Nandrolone, 53
naproxen, 58, 124, 142
narrow therapeutic drugs, 95, 142, 157
nasal sprays, 128
National Poisons Information Service,
    61
nausea, 101, 134
Neo-Mercazole, 30
Neocate Active, 50
nervous tension, 126
neuropathic pain, 112, 150
neurotransmitter dopamine deficiency,
    132
NHS contracts, 98, 144
NHS service standards, 116
Nifedipine, 86
nitrazepam, 33, 136, 167, 179, 190
Nivaquine syrup, 96, 190
nocturia, 12
non-Hodgkin's lymphoma, 18, 56
non-linear pharmacokinetics, 128
non-pharmacy retail outlets, 34
number of charges, 108, 122, 138
nurses, 50, 121, 156
nutritional supplements, 3
Nylax with senna 30 tablets, 34
Nystatin, 150

obesity, 61, 81, 96, 104, 132, 137, 142,
    146
ocular diagnostic preparations, 63
oestradiol hormones, 30
oestrogen-only products, 50
oil of croton, 43
omega-3 content, 87
omeprazole, 30, 122, 124
ondansetron, 29
online pharmacy services, 46, 76
open comedones, 97
operating machinery, 106, 124, 147
opioid-induced constipation, 129
opioids, 77, 123, 124, 134, 137, 159, 193
Opticians Act 1984, 41
optometrists, 121, 156
oral antidiabetic drugs, 112
oral contraceptives, 93, 108, 110, 122,
    134, 149, 155

oral penicillin, 121
oral piroxicam, 45
oral rehydration therapy solution, 14
oral thrush, 97
Order of Malta Ambulance Corps, 41
Orelox tablets, 37
original containers, 32, 35, 61
orlistat, 77, 137
osmotic laxatives, 126
OTC *see* over-the-counter medications
ototoxicity, 142
out-of-pocket expense claims, 27, 62
over-the-counter (OTC) medications,
    21, 119, 128
overdose, 53, 104, 146, 174, 175
OxyContin tablets, 39

P *see* pharmacy-only medicines
pack sizes, 9, 51
package costs, 32
packs, split or broken, 9, 51
pain, 124
    gabapentin, 150
    in legs, 77
    rheumatic disease, 29
    on urinating, 12
Paludrine/Avloclor travel pack, 101
papaveretum, 181, 191
paracetamol, 124, 151, 159, 174
paramedics, 41
parenteral preparations, 15, 41,
    125, 180
Parkinson's Disease, 125, 132
Paroxetine, 134
Part 1 poisons, 75
patient group direction, 43, 112
peanut allergy, 35, 71
pelious hepatitis, 29
penicillamine, 35, 71
penicillin, 43, 121, 124, 156
pentazocine, 39
Peptac, 172, 186
peptic ulcers, 124
percentage strengths, 33, 171
perindopril erbumine, 181
perioperative preparations, 63
peripheral neuropathy, 119, 154
Permitabs, 171, 186
pernicious anaemia, 126
personal and professional conduct, 117

pethidine hydrochloride, 155
pharmacists
    code of ethics, 117
    criminal convictions, 116, 153
    denaturated alcohol, 22
    duties, 21, 24, 45
    personal and professional conduct, 117
    pregnancy test, 99, 144
    supervision, 34
    supplementary prescribers, 112
pharmacodynamics, 109, 149
pharmacokinetics, 109, 128, 132, 149
pharmacy procedure reviews, 76
pharmacy-only (P) medicines, 33, 54, 70,
    113, 151
phenelzine, 121
phenobarbitol, 33, 55, 123, 158
phenothiazines, 145
phenytoin, 128, 133, 146, 155
phosphates, 32
photodynamic treatments, 63
photosensitivity, 59, 138
phototoxicity, 86, 124, 140
phytomenadione, 33
Piperacillin, 49
piperazine phenothiazines, 53
piroxicam, 45, 76
plaque psoriasis, 127
plasma ranges, 72, 132, 173, 187
Plavix, 30
pneumonia, 25, 45
poisons, 14, 26, 75
Polarspeed, 32
polydipsia, 49
POM *see* prescription-only medicines
Ponceau 4R, 52
possession restrictions, 33, 34
potassium chloride, 177
potassium permanganate, 186
potassium replacement therapy, 191
powders, 180
prednisolone, 28, 44, 62, 123, 124, 158,
    170, 185
    side-effects, 28, 102, 110, 158
pregnancy
    antimalarials, 21
    contraindicated drugs, 1, 11, 21
    fetal hypoxia, 31
    folic acid, 84, 139
    safe drugs, 18

tests, 99, 144
tibolone, 47
uterine blood flow, 31
Prempak-C, 44
presciber validity, 98
prescription charges/fees, 7, 9, 80, 90, 122, 140, 157
  exemption from, 107, 148
  number of charges, 44, 108, 122, 138, 157
  *see also* prescriptions
Prescription Intervention Service, 144
prescription-only medicines (POM), 16, 54, 69, 70, 113, 114, 151
  POM-V and POM-VPS, 22
prescriptions, 10, 50
  blacklisted items, 30
  community practitioner nurses, 121
  discounts, 27, 108
  dispensing number of times, 91
  doxycycline, 62
  fraud, 115, 152
  independent nurses, 121
  legal validity, 87
  nurses, 50, 121
  optometrists, 121, 156
  Prempak-C, 44
  SLS reference, 108
  validity, 87, 127, 147, 162
  *see also* prescription charges/fees
preterm babies, 96, 142
preterm neonates, 20
previously administered brand, 119, 154
primary dysmenorrhoea, 58
private prescriptions, 116
procyclidine, 83
professional conduct, 117
prolonged-release formulations, 20, 57
promethazine hydrochloride, 128
propranolol, 32
proprietary preparations, 37
prostate cancer, 29
protein binding, 132
protein content, 3
prothrombin time, 30
Protium tablets, 36
pseudoephedrine tablets, 128
psoriasis, 13
Psorin ointment, 37
psychotic episode, 181

public sale preparations, 28
pulmonary embolism, 32
pulmonary toxicity, 126
Pyrazinamide, 85
pyrexia, 96, 143
Pyridoxine, 56

quality of NHS services, 116
quetiapine, 5
quinalbarbitone, 33, 127
quinine anhydrous base, 86, 170, 185
quinine dihydrochloride, 86, 170, 185
quinine sulphate, 170
quinolones, 44, 140, 145, 163, 164

Raloxifene 60 mg tablets, 51
rate of infusion, 176
rebound congestion, 148
records, 22, 40, 94
Rectogesic rectal ointment, 180
recurrent migraine, 29
red blood cells, 126
red synthetic dyes, 52
red-brown capsules, 31
referrals, 62, 119, 146, 152
refrigeration temperature, 87
registered chiropodists, 33
registered midwifes, 39
reimbursements, 8, 10, 27, 51, 108
religious beliefs, 135, 166
Remedeine tablets, 54
renal failure, 56
renal impairment, 1, 3, 19, 26, 32, 47, 48, 192
repeat prescriptions, 16, 144
reporting
  adverse effects, 52
  to doctors, 20, 101
  error reporting, 24
  faulty medical devices, 100
  indapamide, 11
  to local authority, 25
  urinary problems, 12
requisitions, 23
Resolor, 30
Respimat solution, 62
responsible pharmacist duties, 21, 24, 45
reverse fluid depletion, 143
reviewing pharmacy procedures, 76
rhabdomyolysis, 31

rheumatic disease, 29
rheumatoid arthritis, 131
rhinitis medicamentosa, 107, 148
Rifadin syrup, 37
Rifampicin, 85
right upper quadrant pain, 106
riluzole, 5
rimexolone, 29
ringworm, 147
risperidone orodispersible tablets, 36
rizatriptan, 19
Roaccutane capsules, 25, 35, 71
rosacea, 127
rose water, 179, 190
Rowachol capsules, 37
Royal Pharmaceutical Society's
    guidance, 116
Royal Pharmaceutical Society's
    inspector checks, 114
Sabril, 31
safety phrase labelling, 42
St John's wort, 126
salbutamol, 124, 142, 159
salbutamol base, 170, 186
salbutamol sulphate, 170, 186
saline nasal drops, 128
salmeterol, 126
Salmosan, 42
scabies, 127
schedule 1 controlled drugs, 83, 165
schedule 2 controlled drugs, 23, 40, 93,
    94, 123
schedule 3 controlled drugs, 23, 40, 43,
    123, 165
schedule 4 controlled drugs, 123
schedule 5 controlled drugs, 123
schizophrenia, 84, 118
Scotland, 41
Securon, 31
sedating antihistamines, 128
seizure thresholds, 123, 157
seizures, 32, 33, 44, 163
selected list schemes (SLS), 52, 108
Seretide inhalers, 30
serum concentrations, 120, 155, 175
shelf-lives, 118
sickle-cell anaemia, 126
simvastatin, 86, 140
sitaxentan sodium, 32
skin conditions, 105, 127

skin staining, 35, 71, 145
SLA *see* selected list schemes
sleeping, 12
smooth-muscle relaxants, 15
sodium, 6, 12, 50
sodium bicarbonate, 183, 193
sodium chloride, 95, 172, 177, 184,
    189, 193
sodium fluoride, 93, 182, 188
sodium ions, 172, 186
SOP *see* standard operating procedures
sore throats, 30, 101
Sotalol, 141
SPC *see* Summary of Product
    Characteristics
specification on prescriptions, 106
speech problems, 129
Spiriva, 28
spironolactone, 78, 122, 157
split or broken packages, 9, 51
staining, 35, 71, 145
standard operating procedures (SOP),
    116
standards, 116, 135
statement questions, 39, 131
sterculia granules, 129
stock removal, 39, 99
stockings, 122, 138, 157
storage, 87, 103, 132, 140, 144, 145
Strattera capsules, 35
strong opioids, 123, 159
subcutaneous injections, 183
subtherapeutic levels, 120
Subutex, 116
sucralfate, 36, 72
suicide ideation, 31
Summary of Product Characteristics
    (SPC), 134, 166
sunburn, 86
surgical spirit, 43
Suspected Adverse Reaction Surveillance
    Scheme (SARSS), 22, 58
symbols, 104, 146
Synalar, 35
synthetic dyes, 52
Sytron elixir, 187

tachycardia, 139
Tagamet, 11, 173, 187
tamoxifen, 128

tamsulosin hydrochloride tablets, 103
Tazocin, 5, 49
temazepam, 34, 93, 123, 132, 141, 158, 165
temperature range storage, 87
tendon damage, 44
teratogenics, 4, 36, 48, 52, 60
terbulatine sulphate, 49
tetracycline, 111
thalassaemia major, 126
thalidomide, 48
theophylline, 120, 128
therapeutic dose monitoring, 95, 142, 157
therapeutic drug monitoring, 77, 122, 126, 161
therapeutic effect times, 128
therapeutic range, 128, 132
tiaprofenic acid, 57
tibolone, 3, 47
Tilade, 37
tinidazole, 36
Tinzaparin, 48
tiotropium, 62
topical preparations, 35, 148
toxic overdose, 128
toxicity/toxic effects
    aminoglycoside, 96
    aspirin, 156
    ciclosporin, 72
    classification questions, 129
    digoxin, 83, 104, 138, 139, 145, 146
    gentamicin, 96, 142
    grapefruit juice, 36
    lithium, 164
    vancomycin, 111, 150
trade names, 2, 5, 49
trade-specific denatured alcohol (TSDA), 22
tramadol, 123, 124, 134, 158
tranylcypromine, 36
triamcinolone, 44
tricyclic antidepressants, 81, 138
Tritace, 31
Troch, 96, 143
TSDA *see* trade-specific denatured alcohol
type 2 diabetes, 96, 110, 132, 142
typical absence seizures, 32
tyrosine kinase inhibitors, 31

urinary issues, 12
urinary retention, 138, 139
urinary tract infections, 111, 121, 150
urine discolouration, 30, 80, 124, 137
uterine blood flow, 31
Utinor tablets, 35
Utrogestan capsules, 36

vaccines, 20
vaginal candidiasis, 111
valaciclovir, 29
vancomycin, 111, 150
ventricular arrhythmias, 31
verapamil, 32, 155
vertigo, 125
veterinary preparations, 22, 43, 117, 153
vision, 31, 137, 139, 146
vitamins
    absorption, 148
    vitamin A, 172, 186
    vitamin $B_6$ deficiency, 19, 56
    vitamin $B_{12}$ deficiency, 123, 126, 158
    vitamin D, 107
    vitamin K, 30, 95, 142
vomiting, 101, 134
voriconazole, 18

warfarin, 32, 83, 122, 123, 132, 139
waste regulations, 41, 99
weak opioids, 77, 123, 137, 159
websites, 46, 76
Welldorm tablets, 34
wholesale supplies, 16, 23, 55
withdrawal effects, 32, 123, 158, 164, 166
wound treatments, 30

Xarelto tablets, 34
xerostomia, 20, 58

Yasmin, 122, 149, 157
Yellow Card scheme, 25, 60

Zerit capsules, 37
zidovudine, 181, 191
Zimovane, 52
zinc, 32, 35
zopiclone, 52